THERAPY IN PRACTICE SERIES

Edited by Jo Campling

This series of books is aimed at 'therapists' concerned with rehabilitation in a very broad sense. The intended audience particularly includes occupational therapists, physiotherapists and speech therapists, but many titles will also be of interest to nurses, psychologists, medical staff, social workers, teachers or volunteer workers. Some volumes are interdisciplinary, others are aimed at one particular profession. All titles will be comprehensive but concise, and practical but with due reference to relevant theory and evidence. They are not research monographs but focus on professional practice, and will be of value to both students and qualified personnel.

1. Occupation Therapy for Children with Disabilities
   Dorothy E. Penso
2. Living Skills for Mentally Handicapped People
   Christine Peck and Chia Swee Hong
3. Rehabilitation of the Older Patient
   Edited by Amanda J. Squires
4. Physiotherapy and the Elderly Patient
   Paul Wagstaff and Davis Coakley
5. Rehabilitation of the Severely Brain-Injured Adult
   Edited by Ian Fussey and Gordon Muir Giles
6. Communication Problems in Elderly People
   Rosemary Gravell
7. Occupational Therapy Practice in Psychiatry
   Linda Finlay
8. Working with Bilingual Language Disability
   Edited by Deirdre M. Duncan
9. Counselling Skills for Health Professionals
   Philip Burnard
10. Teaching Interpersonal Skills
    A handbook of experiential learning for health professionals
    Philip Burnard
11. Occupational Therapy for Stroke Rehabilitation
    Simon B. N. Thompson and Maryanne Morgan
12. Assessing Physically Disabled People at Home
    Kathy Maczka
13. Acute Head Injury
    Practical management in rehabilitation
    Ruth Garner
14. Practical Physiotherapy with Older People
    Lucinda Smyth et al.
15. Keyboard, Graphic and Handwriting Skills
    Helping people with motor disabilities
    Dorothy E. Penso

16. Community Occupational Therapy with Mentally Handicapped Adults
   Debbie Isaac
17. Autism
   Professional perspectives and practice
   Edited by Kathryn Ellis
18. Multiple Sclerosis
   Approaches to management
   Edited by Lorraine De Souza
19. Occupational Therapy in Rheumatology
   An holistic approach
   Lynne Sandles
20. Breakdown of Speech
   Causes and remediation
   Nancy R. Milloy
21. Coping with Stress in the Health Professions
   A practical guide
   Philip Burnard
22. Speech and Communication Problems in Psychiatry
   Rosemary Gravell and Jenny France
23. Limb Amputation
   From aetiology to rehabilitation
   Rosalind Ham and Leonard Cotton
24. Management in Occupational Therapy
   Zielfa B. Maslin
25. Rehabilitation in Parkinson's Disease
   Francis Caird

Coping with Stress in the Health Professions

A practical guide

PHILIP BURNARD

Lecturer, University of Wales College of Medicine, Cardiff, Wales
Honorary Lecturer, Institute for Higher Professional Education for
Health Care Professions, Hogeschool Midden Nederland, Utrecht,
The Netherlands

CHAPMAN & HALL
London · New York · Tokyo · Melbourne · Madras

UK	Chapman & Hall, 2–6 Boundary Row, London SE1 8HN
USA	Chapman & Hall, 29 West 35th Street, New York NY10001
JAPAN	Chapman & Hall Japan, Thomson Publishing Japan, Hirakawacho Nemoto Building, 7F, 1–7–11 Hirakawa-cho, Chiyoda-ku, Tokyo 102
AUSTRALIA	Chapman & Hall Australia, Thomas Nelson Australia, 102 Dodds Street, South Melbourne, Victoria 3205
INDIA	Chapman & Hall India, R. Seshadri, 32 Second Main Road, CIT East, Madras 600 035

First edition 1991

© 1991 P. Burnard

Phototypeset in 10/12 Times by Input Typesetting Ltd, London
Printed in Great Britain by St Edmundsbury Press Ltd,
Bury St Edmunds, Suffolk

ISBN 0 412 38910 X

British Library Cataloguing in Publication Data
Burnard, Philip
  Coping with stress in the health professions.
  1. Medical personnel. Stress
  I. Title
  610.69019

  ISBN 0–412–38910–X

Library of Congress Cataloging-in-Publication Data available

For Les, Paul, Mark and Ian

Contents

Acknowledgements   x

Preface   xi

1. Stress and the health professional   1
2. Stress and feelings   15
3. Stress and self-awareness   32
4. Self-awareness activities for stress   62
5. Stress and relaxation   76
6. Stress, values and meditation   86
7. Stress and assertiveness   98
8. Stress and its effects on you   111
9. Stress support systems for individuals   122
10. Group support and supervision   149

Appendix   169

References   171

Bibliography   176

Index   188

Acknowledgements

This is not just a book about stress. It is a book about coping with stress in the health professions. I am very grateful to a number of social workers, nurses, physiotherapists, occupational therapists, teachers and students who have told me what they find stressful in their work and how they cope with stress themselves. I have used much of this information in the form of direct quotes and as composite case studies. My thanks go to: Irmgard Bauer, J. Bonsall, Liz Brown, Ian Chesterfield, Elizabeth Ingram, Tim Kilner, Sandy Kirkman, Sinead Lodge, Rosie Morton, John Pugh, Annie Rae, A. Thomas, and all the people who have helped me.

Thanks, too, to my colleague and friend, Paul Morrison – particularly for his discussion on the issue of *caring* in the health professions.

As always, I am grateful to Jo Campling for her guidance and editorial advice.

Acknowledgement is given to Pergamon Press, Oxford, for permission to use the Holmes–Rahe Social Readjustment Rating Scale. Acknowledgement is also given to Meg Bond of the Human Potential Resource Group, University of Surrey, Guildford, for permission to quote from J. Heron's 1981 Paradigm Papers, in Chapter 1.

Most of all, thanks go to my family: my wife, Sally, and my children, Aaron and Rebecca, who have been patient and supportive throughout the project.

Preface

Stress is a feature of all of our lives. The business of working in the health professions means that we are constantly being exposed to stress. That stress can sometimes be enriching and motivating. It has often been pointed out that stress can be positive or negative. When stress is positive, it rarely needs any further attention. When it is negative, it is a problem.

The first aim of this book is to discuss the various sorts of stress that may be experienced by a variety of health professionals, including social workers, nurses, doctors, physiotherapists, occupational therapists and others. What they all have in common is that they work closely with other people – people who often have emotional problems or problems in living. Working with other people who are troubled in this way is indeed stressful. For too long it has been assumed that health professionals should 'get on with it' and put up with any stress that is involved in caring for others.

The second aim of this book is to offer practical ways of coping with negative stress. These methods range from simple relaxation techniques, through meditation to methods that involve discussing stress with others: counselling, co-counselling and group work.

All the methods described in this book have been used with a variety of health professionals, and not all of these methods will necessarily appeal to you. One of the fundamental points about stress is that it tends to affect each individual idiosyncratically. Therefore it seems reasonable to suppose that methods of combating stress will vary from person to person, and it will be to our advantage if some of the methods are tested. The danger when we are stressed is not only the stress itself, but the fact that we do nothing about it. The methods here are simple and straightforward and rarely take much time.

What this book is *not* is a detailed research monograph on stress. Many excellent books of that sort have already been written and the reader is referred to many of those in the accompanying bibliography. More than anything, I hope that this book is *practical*. In doing the research for the book I have been fortunate in having had the help of a wide range health professionals who have told me what they find stressful about their profession and how they cope with stress. Wherever possible I have tried to incorporate those factors into the book and they have guided me in what to include and what to leave out. Health professionals care for others all the time. I hope that this book can enable some to care more for themselves. It was enjoyable to write; I hope it is easy to read. I would welcome any comments you have about it.

PHILIP BURNARD
University of Wales College of Medicine,
Cardiff

1

Stress and the health professional

What is stress? You can't see it but you know its there. I would say it's the alternative to success. There's only a thin line between swimming and sinking with the fear of drowning always evident. As a student, I'm still splashing about out there . . .

Student physiotherapist

Aims of this chapter

This chapter explores:

- The nature of stress
- The causes of stress
- Stress and health professionals
- Examples from practice
- Stress and burnout.

THE NATURE OF STRESS

All health professionals experience stress. The very fact of caring for others – in whatever capacity – means that we are open to suffering from stress and stress-related problems. The aim of this book is a practical one: to offer ways of coping with stress. While it is acknowledged that we should all be working to make our jobs less stressful and to deal with the issues *behind* the stress, the fact is that all the time we have to cope. Studs Terkel, the American researcher and journalist, summed up the nature of stress related to working with others (Terkel, 1972) when he wrote that:

> work is, by its very nature, about violence . . . to the spirits as well as to the body. It is about ulcers as well as accidents, about shouting matches as well as fistfights, about nervous breakdowns as well as kicking the dog around. It is, above all (or beneath all), about daily humiliations. To survive the day is triumph enough for the walking wounded among the great many of us.

Stress in Health Care: a Case in Point   1

Lloyd Webster is a thirty-year old social worker who has a heavy case load in a difficult area of south London. He finds that he tends to 'take his work home with him' and this is beginning to affect his home life. He and his wife frequently argue, especially about the fact that he seems to talk about little but work.

Lloyd's wife reads about methods of time management and organization and suggests that Lloyd be allowed to talk about work only for a particular period each day, on return from work. She encourages Lloyd to plan his work more carefully so that he does not feel so pressurized. The fact that the couple have talked about a difficult problem in both of their lives means that the pressure is taken out of the situation and both begin to relax more easily. As a result, too, both Lloyd and his wife begin to communicate with each other more clearly.

Stress in Health Care: a Case in Point   2

Sarah is a student nurse working in a psychiatric hospital. Because she is new to the job, she has trouble expressing to the people she works with how difficult she finds working in clinical settings. Her second allocation, to an acute unit, is particularly arduous. During a period in the college of nursing, Sarah learns about assertiveness. As a result, she learns both to express how she feels about her job and also learns to say 'no' to what she perceives as excessive demands being made of her by her colleagues.

Many of us in the health professions are among the walking

wounded. We have to live, we have to care for others, we have to cope. This book, then, is about the process of coping.

What we need, to start with, is a working definition of stress. Various commentators have defined stress in different ways (see, for example Cox, 1978b; Bailey and Clarke, 1989, etc.). It is defined here as *psychological, physiological and/or spiritual discomfort that is experienced when environmental stimuli are too demanding or exceed a person's coping strategies.* The environmental stimuli alluded to in this definition may range from those that have their source in our immediate surroundings, those that are caused by other people or those that are within us. We never have an occasion when we are *not* responding to stimuli, and stress can be caused by 'stimulus overload', or sometimes by lack of stimuli, or by inappropriate stimuli. It is notable, too, that stress has been classified in various ways. In the following section, three broad approaches are explored briefly.

APPROACHES TO STRESS

Bailey and Clarke (1989) identify three approaches to stress:

1. Stress can be defined as something, outside the person, to which he or she reacts. In this model, for example, bad lighting or disturbing life events can be examples of stress: the person *responds* to that stress by experiencing *strain*. The problem with this approach is that it tends to treat the person as a passive respondent to stress. Bailey and Clarke call this the *stimulus-based model.*
2. Almost the opposite to the stimulus-based model is the *response-based* approach. Here, stress is used to denote a person's physiological response to a difficult environment or distressing life event. Perhaps the best-known example of this approach is Hans Selye's General Adaptation Syndrome (Selye, 1956, 1975). Selye (1975) defines the stress syndrome as 'the non-specific response of the body to any demand made upon it'. Stress, for Selye, causes physiological changes in the body and a whole range of stressors can cause similar sorts of physiological responses.
3. The mid-position between these two is the *transactional model of stress.* This model acknowledges that an individual's *perception* of a situation plays a large part in determining whether or

not that situation is stressful, and takes into account the fact that different people find different situations stressful at different points in their lives. The person in this model is neither a passive recipient of stress nor a consistent responder to it, but instead responds to difficult life events via his or her idiosyncratic *coping style*. This is more *psychological* than the two previous approaches.

The first two of these approaches to stress tend to favour a physiological view of stress: stressful events occur and the body responds accordingly. The last, more psychological approach, acknowledges that individuals respond differently to a variety of stimuli. What causes a stress response in one person may spur another on. Arguably, it is difficult to lay down 'typical' stress responses: everything, it would seem, is dependent upon *this* individual's history, expectations, physical and psychological status and previous experience. The approach taken in this book is that it is important for **you** to identify **your** ways of coping and **your** ways of dealing with stress. By becoming more self-aware it is possible to notice your reactions and to choose what to do about them. That choice is broadened by having knowledge of a range of possible ways of coping. This book offers such a range.

SOURCES OF STRESS

John Heron (1981) offers what he calls a 'comprehensive account of sources of human stress'. They are:

- Foetal experience and the primal experiences approaching, during and after birth.
- The frustration of and interference with physical and psychological needs in early infancy and childhood, with residual lifelong effects.
- The frustration of and interference with physical and psychological needs in present time, in adulthood.
- Conflicts arising within the interpretation and expression of a given or adopted social role; and between different social roles a person has.
- Constraints due to oppressive organizational structures and procedures (from the family, through the work organization, to the State).

- Stress to do with certain basic features of the human condition that interact with all the above items:

  - the phenomenon of human separation; through birth, partings, death;
  - the tension between survival needs and needs for personal and cultural fulfilment;
  - ignorance, lack of knowledge: the apparent inscrutability of many phenomena;
  - the intractability of matter and the world; the frustrating gap between the ideal and actuality between vision and its realization;
  - the inherent instability of human beings' vast but unprogrammed potential; the tension and stress due to the very plethora of choice and possibility for persons;
  - the presence of other persons subject to all the stresses of the same conditions.

- Pressures, interferences and constraints due to the unseen climate, to what is going in the other reality and its incursion into the human realm.
- Being eccentric, off centre, alienated and disassociated from one's source and origin.

Heron's list seems almost overwhelming in its coverage of the possible sources of stress in the individual. The list ranges from the factors of being alive, through the problems associated with our relationships with ourselves and with others and on to spiritual notions of 'other realities' and of the sheer unpredictability and intractability of much of what is happening in the world. It also identifies the problems associated with the differences between what we *want* to do and what we *can* do. All of these issues will be familiar in one form or another to the health professional. The items in the list may apply either to the health professional's clients, to the health professional personally, or to both : they are the basic stressors of everyday living.

STRESS AND HEALTH PROFESSIONALS

Various stressors of health professionals have been identified in the literature. A number of writers describe the stress of health professionals fighting against time pressures and having to make

5

instant decisions that may affect patient care (Firth and Shapiro, 1986). One radiography teacher suggested:

> The most stressful aspect of being a radiographer is working alone and being extremely busy. I have to prioritize examinations and therefore delay the radiography of patients. I have to cope with many situations at the same time, attempting to meet several deadlines . . .

A metaphor that is sometimes used to convey this pressure of work and limit of time relates it to a person rescuing people from a raging river but being unable to stop and go further up river to see what is causing the people to fall in.

All health professionals face occupational hazards of various sorts. Apart from the problems associated with possible disease and infection, Margison (1987), Jones (1987) and Rushton (1987) suggest that those working in psychiatry and social work face the added stressor of possible violence. Clearly, working in an atmosphere in which there is a threat of personal attack is likely to cause anxiety and stress reactions.

Managing in times of cutback and financial restraint also clearly causes stress. More than ever before, the health professions face stringent times, which often means that they have to face situations for which they are ill-prepared. As one lecturer in nursing studies put it: 'I am constantly being put into new situations where my knowledge is insufficient and I have to play things by ear . . .'

Jick (1987) offers the following techniques for improving effectiveness in the health professions in times of budget cuts:

- Maximize downward communication.
- Involve affected parties as much as possible.
- Reshape expectation levels to sustain motivation.
- Build on readiness to make cuts, not resistance.
- Provide outlets for stress release.
- Be prepared to take some grief.

In his last item, Jick acknowledges that administrators must be prepared to listen to the voicing of hostile feelings and complaints from subordinates who are suffering the effects of cutbacks. Thus, in turn, the health professional administrator is also subject to stress.

Patients and clients can be sources of stress. The process of caring for such a range of people with such a variety of problems and emotions can often be particularly stressful. A nurse complained of:

. . . mental 'leap-frogging' – one minute sad, sympathetic and passive, the next minute welcoming, approachable, friendly. Too much of this chopping and changing in a day is exhausting.

Caring for others can often lead to self-neglect. John Heron has described the problem of the 'compulsive carer' (Heron, 1975) – the person who *has* to look after others. Sometimes this compulsion leads to a lack of assertion and an inability to refuse others' requests. A nurse tutor stated:

I have to be careful to say 'no' sometimes, when asked to do things. I find saying 'no' difficult. When I have committed myself to many things I find these tend to play on my mind.

At other times, the process of coping with the extremes of emotions causes stress. One ward sister suggested that it was stressful to have to

. . . break bad news to people I feel I don't know very well . . . for example, telling relatives of a new admission that their relative may not recover.

Sometimes, organizational constraints cause stress. A lecturer in midwifery said that she found it stressful.

. . . not knowing whether courses I am designing will be funded or not . . . not knowing if political moves will alter the nature of my work.

These are just some of the ways in which health professionals experience stress in their roles as carers. The long-term effects of stress can build up and cause the syndrome that has been called 'burnout.'

STRESS AND BURNOUT

One particular sort of stress that has been described in the literature is *burnout*. The term is normally used to describe the feelings associated with long-term, job-related stress. Maslach (1981) suggests that:

> Burnout is a syndrome of emotional exhaustion, depersonalization, and reduced personal accomplishment that can occur among individuals who do 'people work' of some kind. It is a response to the chronic emotional strain of dealing extensively with other human beings, particularly when they are troubled or having problems. Thus, it can be considered one type of job stress.

Burnout is usually associated with working in caring professions, under considerable stress, for long periods. Characteristics include:

- Loss of motivation.
- The development of negative rather than positive attitudes towards the job and towards other people.
- The development of a 'gallows' sense of humour or a loss of sense of humour altogether.
- A sense of a narrowing choice of options.
- A feeling that one is acted upon rather than exercising choice.

Levine (1982) sums up both the problem of burnout and a dubious solution to it, thus:

> There is an ancient joke about psychotherapists which long preceded today's concern about alienation and burnout. A young analyst, frazzled at the end of each day's emotional wear and tear, enviously observed an older, more experienced colleague who seemed to leave the office at the end of each day fresh and carefree. Screwing up his courage, the younger man finally asked his more experienced colleague, 'How can you leave the office so full of energy, and so fresh after listening to all of your patients' troubles all day long?' The older man looked at his younger colleague and said, 'Who listens?'

Perhaps many health professionals cope only by stopping listening either to their clients or to themselves.

Maslach (1976) identifies three stages in the process of burnout: (1) emotional exhaustion, (2) depersonalization and (3) feelings of reduced personal accomplishment.

Emotional exhaustion

As we have noted, caring for others can be a stressful business. The first characteristic of the onset of burnout is a sense of emotional fatigue. The carer feels that he or she has little left to give to others and begins to cope with this by gradually cutting away from others. This leads to stage two, the stage of depersonalization.

Depersonalization

In this stage, the fact of cutting oneself off from others as a coping strategy leads to a sense of alienation from others. Others are also viewed in a negative light and the health professional often begins, actively, to dislike those people who were previously cared for or worked with. It is not uncommon to hear health professionals remark in a cynical way, 'the job would be O.K. if it weren't for the clients . . .' for the person experiencing burnout, this sentiment becomes a reality. Often the person expends a lot of energy in trying to avoid clients and others. Sometimes this is through burying himself or herself in paperwork and administration. Sometimes it is by keeping appointments very brief. Overall, the feeling is one of negative attitudes towards self and others.

Reduced personal accomplishment

All of this distancing takes its toll. The persons experiencing burnout end up by feeling that very little is being achieved. In some cases this is true; in others, the negative attitudes lead to an inability to self-assess and to evaluate work outcomes. Sometimes, all past work is 'rubbished'. The burntout persons start to feel that *nothing* he or they have done in the field of caring has been worthwhile and that if they had previously viewed themselves as caring, they had been deluded. It is at this point that many people choose to leave the profession and seek work in a situation where they can avoid others. Others learn to cope by adopting a distant or cynical approach towards other people. So what can be done?

COPING WITH BURNOUT

Pines, Aronson and Kafry (1981) suggest four major strategies for coping with burnout:

- Being aware of the problem.
- Taking responsibility for doing something about it.
- Achieving some degree of cognitive clarity.
- Developing new skills for coping.

Practical Methods of Coping with Stress in the Health Professions: 1

POSTURE

Take time to notice your posture. Do you tend to hunch your shoulders or to drop your head as you sit or walk? If so, notice your posture and make small adjustments to make yourself more comfortable. Stress often shows itself in the ways that we sit, walk and move.

Being aware of the problem

The first stage must be the recognition that a problem exists. This is not always easy as the process of burnout is often so insidious. Sometimes the change of attitude in the person experiencing burnout is noted by a colleague and this offers the chance for discussion of the problem. Even then, it is common for burnout people to deny that anything is wrong or, if there is, to see the problem as being *external* to themselves. Very often, a person's distress is displaced onto the job, the organization or onto other people. Thus it is not uncommon for people suffering from this type of stress reaction to claim that the organization 'no longer cares' for them, or that 'the job has changed and isn't interesting any more'. Rarely can the person 'own' the problem and identify that while the job and the clients have contributed to burnout, the problem lies within. This recognition must occur if something is to change.

Taking responsibility for doing something about it

Linked to identifying that a problem exists is the recognition that, if anything is to change, the person with burnout must take the initiative in doing something about it. Unfortunately, this is usually what the person feels least able to do. He or she often feels powerless and demotivated to the point of merely being able to struggle through. This is where help from other colleagues and friends can make a difference. Through talking through the issues and through being heard by another person, the carer with burnout can reach the decision to change his or her situation.

Achieving some degree of cognitive clarity

Burnout has a distinct emotional component. As we have noted, the burnout person often feels trapped and disinterested. The point, in this stage, is to carefully itemize *exactly* what the issues are that are contributing to the state of burnout. It is never only the case that a person feels emotionally exhausted. Things are happening to those people to make them feel that way. A careful analysis of what is happening in the person's life and work can lead to the identification of solutions. For example, at a workshop on coping with burnout, a staff nurse identified the following issues that contributed to her burntout feeling:

- Working too long in one clinical area.
- Doing two jobs: one at the NHS hospital and private work for a nursing agency.
- Not having attended any further education courses or workshops for over two years.
- Not facing up to a clash of personalities between her and a colleague.

As a result of identifying these issues, she was able to set clearly defined aims, as follows:

- Make appointment to see nurse manager about a change of ward.
- Cut down on private nursing and aim towards working at one job only.
- Write for an Open University Prospectus, read nursing journals and look for a course to undertake over the following months.
- Attend a local assertiveness course, which should enable her to confront her colleague.

Developing new skills for coping

The process of gaining cognitive clarity leads to the development of ways of coping with burnout. Nothing else alters unless a behavioural change occurs. The first stage in achieving such behavioural change is the identification of clear objectives, as noted above. This is not to suggest that *everything* that contributes to a person feeling burnout can be changed, but to suggest that, with clear goals, some things *can* be changed. The point about such goals is that they need to be clearly stated and achievable.

HOW HEALTH PROFESSIONALS COPE WITH STRESS

Just as stress affects people in numerous ways, so the mechanisms for coping with it can be various. Here are some of the ways that health professionals of a variety of disciplines – ranging from physiotherapists to nurses and from radiographers to occupational therapists – cope with stress:

- I remind myself of the supportive network which I value alot – colleagues, friends and family. Then I don't feel alone.
- I am learning to say 'no'. When I am stressed about things, I use diversion. I tell myself that things are not so important.
- I listen to music, watch TV or play with the children.
- I talk about the situation either with a close friend in the profession or with my superior.
- I throw something at the wall!
- I find doing physical things, like running and circuit training, to be very helpful.

- The only way I see of my coping with stress is to extinguish the causes.
- I find it helps having a spiritual life and friends from the church to sympathize effectively.
- I enjoy laughing immoderately!
- I find it helpful to talk things through: sometimes with one or two people I feel I can be very frank and honest with; on other occasions I just talk about it to anyone.
- In my mind, I deliver wonderful speeches concerning the matter that I am stressed about!
- I read novels, plays, poetry.
- I make a list of everything that needs to be done and of what is bothering me. If possible, I work down this list before going to bed and tick them off.
- I attend a weekly yoga group and try to practise at home as well.
- Being with my four-year-old stepson reduces my stress – I hadn't realized the richness of experience to be gained from seeing the world through his eyes!
- I play very loud music and lock myself away on my own.
- I cope by trying to switch off completely from work.
- My main source of coping is to go out riding my pony across the moors. It doesn't matter at all about the weather – I always find I feel 're-charged' afterwards.
- I try to do something physical such as swimming, weight training or running.

OTHER APPROACHES TO STRESS

Finally, it is acknowledged that the methods discussed here are only some of the ways that stress may be addressed. Vingerhoets and Marcelissen (1988) have identified nine main approaches to stress research:

1. Biological, e.g. neurological/hormonal response.
2. Psychosomatic, e.g. personality and its role in ill-health.
3. Life events, e.g. the relationship of life events to illness.
4. Transactional, e.g. the study of coping.
5. Life styles, e.g. examining stress-inducing behaviours.
6. Group differences, e.g. comparing men with women.

7. Culture, e.g. its role in the incidence and evidence of stress.
8. Organizational, e.g. the effect of work conditions on stress.
9. Intervention/prevention, e.g. considering management strategies at the person, environmental and societal level.

These strategies cover the whole span of human experience: biological, psychological, sociological, cultural and so forth. While this book cannot address all these factors with equal weight, they all impinge on the way that the health professionals experience their work and themselves. Hopefully, too, the practical activities suggested in this book also address many, if not all, of these aspects.

SUMMARY

This chapter has explored the notion of stress as it relates to health professionals. It has acknowledged the vast array of factors, both internal and external to the person, that can lead to the experience of being unable to cope – sometimes to the point of experiencing burnout.

2

Stress and feelings

One way of describing the way I feel would be to think of yourself in the sea, with the water just lapping at your shoulders. Then, following a couple of hectic days and what seems like a mountain of work to do, you sink a few inches until the water is touching your chin.

Student physiotherapist

Aims of this chapter

This chapter explores:

- The nature of emotions
- Mental mechanisms
- The effects of bottling up emotions
- Positive ways of coping with emotions
- Releasing bottled up emotions.

Stress is often closely related to feelings. We bottle them up, we forget them, we have difficulty in expressing them or we express them in great abundance. While stress affects different people in different ways, it seems that we often feel very stressed because we cannot cope with our emotions.

THE NATURE OF EMOTIONS

John Heron (1977) distinguishes between at least four types of emotion that are commonly suppressed or bottled up: anger, fear,

15

grief and embarrassment. He notes a relationship between these feelings and certain overt expressions of them. Thus, in the stressed person, anger may be expressed as loud sound, fear as trembling, grief through tears and embarrassment by laughter. He notes, also, a relationship between those feelings and certain basic human needs. Heron argues that we all have the need to understand and know what is happening to us. If that knowledge is not forthcoming, we may experience fear. We also need to make choices in our lives, and if those choices are restricted in certain ways, we may feel anger. Thirdly, we need to experience the expression of love and of being loved. If that love is denied to us or is taken from us, we may experience grief. To Heron's basic human needs may be added the need for self-respect and dignity. If such dignity is denied to us, we may feel self-conscious and embarrassed. Practical examples of how these relationships 'work' in everyday life and in the health professions may be illustrated as follows:

> It helps if I can talk to somebody close to me. Sometimes I find that I am very mixed up and then I 'turn off' . . . I don't seem to care any more.

> I remember reaching the point where I was very angry with my patients . . . I obviously couldn't tell them . . . it was irrational really.

> Sometimes I feel very mixed up . . . I become so stressed that I don't know whether to laugh or cry.

In the last example it may be noted how emotions that are suppressed are rarely only of one sort. Very often, bottled-up emotion is a mixture of anger, fear, embarrassment and grief. Often, too, the causes of such blocked emotion are unclear and lost in the history of the person. What is perhaps more important is that the expression of pent-up emotion is often helpful in that it seems to allow the person to be clearer in his or her thinking once it has been expressed. It is as though the blocked emotion 'gets in the way' and its release acts as a means of helping the person to clarify any thoughts or feelings. It is notable that the suppression of feelings can lead to certain problems in living that may be clearly identified. We shall note, later in this chapter, the effects that pent-up emotion can have. Before that, however, it is important to explore how another way of dealing with unpleasant feelings and thoughts is to deny them in certain respects. Here, the concept of mental mechanisms is useful.

Stress in Health Care: a Case in Point 3

The staff in an intensive care unit in a busy district general hospital find that they are increasingly under pressure and are frequently arguing with each other. The senior charge nurse, who has had previous group experience while working as a psychiatric nurse, suggests the setting up of a staff support group.

At first, a number of members of staff are both cynical about the group and suspicious of the charge nurse's motives for setting it up. After three months, however, most of the staff begin to appreciate the facility for talking openly about their feelings about each other and about the patients. One staff nurse does not enjoy the group but benefits, vicariously, from the more relaxed atmosphere that develops in the unit as a result of the support group.

MENTAL MECHANISMS

None of us can accept too much reality. The truth is often painful. Therefore, we learn to cushion ourselves against the truth by the use of what have been called 'mental mechanisms'. These are usually associated with Freud (Hall, 1954), although other writers have also developed his original formulation. Mental mechanisms help us to guard against excessive anxiety and stress by allowing us some breathing space from the truth either about the way the world is or about the way others think or feel about us. Used sparingly, mental mechanisms are healthy – they can save us considerable, unnecessary pain and anguish. On the other hand, their over-use can mean that we are taking avoiding action too often. The other problem arises when we are *unable* to use them – when we see the truth only too clearly. This, too, is a recipe for pain and distress. Some would argue that an inability to use mental mechanisms leads to severe psychological breakdown. What, then, are examples of mental mechanisms?

Projection

Projection refers to the process whereby we see qualities in others that are our own, but of which we are unaware. Consider, for example, the following description of one social worker by another:

> She's a very good social worker . . . its just that she has such a high opinion of herself . . . she always wants to talk about herself and never wants to listen to other people.

Now this *may* be an accurate description of the other person. Alternatively, it may say more about the commentator than it ever does about the person being described. When we describe other people we are frequently offering a description of ourselves. Try this simple exercise:

> Write down the names of four people, two of whom you like and two you dislike. Now write a brief description of each of them. When you have done that, read those descriptions as *descriptions of yourself*. To what degree does the notion of projection show true here? How much of the descriptions related to *them* and how much related to *yourself*?

Notice, in further conversations, any tendency you have to project in this way. Note, too, that it is possible to project feelings on to the environment around us. Take, for example, the person who enters a pub and says, 'This place has an interesting atmosphere.' Arguably, places do not have 'atmospheres' in this context. Instead, we bring the 'atmosphere' with us and project our own thoughts, preferences and feelings onto different environments. Thus the person who is describing a pub in this way is possibly projecting his or her own wishes and desires onto it.

Projection also happens in groups. The group members who constantly talk of the group's 'hostility' may often be projecting their own hostility onto the group. Rather than face that personal hostility, it is safer to discover it in the world around them (i.e. the group). To take this a stage further, some find their own hostility so hard to bear that they project it onto the world at large. Thus they tend to see the world in general as a hostile place. In this case, the lives of those individuals are directed by the notion of the world being hostile. A moments thought would reveal that, in literal terms, the 'world' *cannot* be 'hostile'.

As with all mental mechanisms, it is important to note two possibilities:

(1) that projection is being used; *or*
(2) that the person who is apparently projecting is, in fact, offering a literal description of another person or thing.

Thus, to take the group example, the person who sees the group as 'hostile' may be either projecting his or her own feelings or identifying what is actually happening in the group. It would be unwise to see all human action and description as examples of the use of mental mechanisms. The secret and the skill both lie in being able to differentiate between mental mechanisms and 'the truth'. The safest way of proceeding is possibly to avoid interpreting other people's utterances as mental mechanisms and to concentrate, instead, on our own motives and behaviours. Thus it is helpful for me to be able to identify when I am projecting feelings on to others. It is less helpful (and arguably impossible with any accuracy) for me to observe others doing it. Noticing my own tendency to project can help me to gain self-awareness and can aid in lowering stress levels by slowly coming to *face* the world rather than escape from it.

Rationalization

Rationalization occurs when a rational excuse is offered for behaviour or situations that are otherwise painful to accept. Consider this example of a student nurse who opens the letter stating that he or she has failed the final examinations:

> I don't care really . . . anyway, no one could pass an examination after the training *we* had. No one ever helped you to get through exams.

Again, as with projection, two things *could* be happening here. The student could be rationalizing the true feelings of disappointment at receiving bad news. Alternatively, he or she could be expressing truths about the training in the reactions to failing the exam! Again, it may be more helpful to notice your own tendency to rationalize in this way than it is to observe the possible rationalization of others.

A degree of rationalization helps us to avoid considerable anxiety, especially in the short term. In the long run, however, it is probably better that we learn to accept things as they really are and to avoid offering 'excuses' for what we do or feel. Identifying a tendency to rationalize excessively can be part of the process of becoming self-aware and such self-awareness can, in the long term, help us to reduce stress.

Reaction-formation

Reaction-formation is a rather different sort of mental mechanism. It is the process by which we sometimes express *exactly the opposite* feeling to the one that we really hold. Consider, for example, the young man who moans about another and who says that if he met him, he would tell him exactly what he thinks of him. Consider, too, when the pair meet and the one who has been moaning greets the other with: 'Hello David: its good to see you again! How are you keeping?' This is one example of reaction-formation. Arguably what is happening here is that it is safer for the person to stay amicable with the other rather than face a showdown with the person he dislikes.

A deeper and perhaps more sinister example of reaction-formation occurs when a person has a deep-seated anxiety about one aspect of his or her personality and deals with this by berating anyone else that has this personality aspect. Consider, for example, the person who 'hates' homosexuals and takes every opportunity to express that hatred while constantly denying personal homosexual tendencies.

Again, it is possible to see the value of identifying our own tendencies towards reaction-formation. If we can identify the 'opposites' that exist within us we can learn to know ourselves better. We can begin to appreciate that many of our prejudices and dislikes are related to ourselves.

Intellectualization

Intellectualization is a defence against emotion. The person who intellectualizes is the one who constantly seeks a rational answer to everything rather than allowing some things to be 'felt' rather than 'known'. The educational systems in the West have typically favoured rationality above the emotions and it is hardly surprising, therefore, that many people have a tendency to want logical explanations for events, behaviours and thoughts. The person who intellectualizes, however, *over-uses* the logical sense and uses it to avoid having to face emotion.

Jung (1978) argued that the mind has at least four functions: thinking, feeling, sensing and intuiting. He also suggested that the emotionally balanced person is the one who can make use of all four functions. The person who intellectualizes will tend to use the thinking and sensing modes in preference to the feeling and intuitive. It is possible, too, that such a person will soon irritate others by the insistent use of and appeal to logic. Not everything in the human condition, after all, can be explained in this way. In the caring professions, it is important that we come to know our emotional side as well as our more rational. Arguably, too, the person who only deals with life on an intellectual plane will bottle up emotional feelings in the way described elsewhere in this chapter. It is perhaps healthier to be aware of our feelings as well as our intellect.

THE EFFECTS OF BOTTLING-UP EMOTIONS

In the discussions so far, we have considered the nature of the emotions and the ways in which we sometimes delude ourselves in order to save ourselves further stress and discomfort. What, then, are the long- and short-term effects of bottling-up emotions?

Physical discomfort and muscular pain

Wilhelm Reich, a psychoanalyst with a particular interest in the relationship between emotions and the musculature, noted that blocked emotions could become trapped in the body's muscle clusters (Reich, 1949). Thus he noted that anger was frequently 'trapped' in the muscles of the shoulders, grief in muscles surrounding the stomach and fear in the leg muscles. Often, these trapped emotions lead to chronic postural problems. Sometimes, the thorough release of the blocked emotion can lead to a freeing of the muscles and an improved physical appearance. Reich believed in working directly on the muscle clusters in order to bring about emotional release and subsequent freedom from suppression, and from his work was developed a particular type of mind/body therapy, known as 'bioenergetics' (Lowen, 1967; Lowen and Lowen, 1977).

Trapped emotion is sometimes 'visible' in a client's posture, and the skilled professional can learn to notice tension in the musculature and changes in breathing patterns that may suggest muscular tension. We have noted throughout this text how difficult it is to interpret another person's behaviour. What is important, here, is that such bodily manifestations be used only as a clue to what may be happening in the person. We cannot assume that a person who looks tense is tense, until that person has said that he or she is under stress.

Health professionals will be very familiar with the link between body posture, the musculature and the emotional state of the person. Frequently, if patients and clients can be helped to relax, then their medical and psychological condition may improve more quickly. Those health professionals who deal most directly with the muscle clusters (remedial gymnasts and physiotherapists, for example) will tend to notice physical tension more readily but all carers can train themselves to observe these important indicators of the emotional status of the person in their care.

Difficulty in decision-making

This is a frequent side effect of bottled-up emotion. It is as though the emotion makes the person uneasy and that uneasiness leads to a lack of confidence. As a result, that person finds it difficult to rely on his or her own resources and may find decision-making difficult. When we are under stress of any sort, it is often the case that we feel the need to check decisions with other people. Once some of this stress is removed by talking through problems or by releasing pent-up emotions, the decision-making process often becomes easier.

Faulty self-image

When we suppress feelings, those feelings often have an unpleasant habit of turning against us. Thus, instead of expressing anger towards others, we turn it against ourselves and feel depressed as a result. Or, if we have hung onto unexpressed grief, we turn that grief in on ourselves and experience ourselves as less than we are. Often, as old resentments or dissatisfactions are expressed, during counselling, the person begins to feel better about his or her self-image.

Setting unrealistic goals

Tension can lead to further tension. This tension can lead us to set ourselves unattainable targets – as though we had set ourselves up to fail! Sometimes, too, failing is a way of punishing ourselves, or it is 'safer' than achieving. Release of tension, through the expression of emotion, can sometimes lead an individual to taking a more realistic view of his or her personality and ambitions.

The development of long-term faulty beliefs

Sometimes, emotion that has been suppressed for a long time can lead to a person's view of the world being coloured in a particular way. The person learns that 'people can't be trusted' or 'people always let you down in the end'. It is as though old, painful feelings lead to distortions that become part of that person's world-view. Such long-term distorted beliefs about the world do not change easily, but may be modified as the individual learns to release feelings and handle personal emotions more effectively.

Practical Methods of Coping with Stress in the Health Professions: 2

BREATHING

Pay attention to your breathing. For a few moments, breathe in through your nose and out through your mouth. Allow your breaths to deepen and allow your stomach to relax as you breathe in. As you breathe out, pull your stomach muscles in a little, to aid exhalation. Begin to notice how you breathe at work, when you get tense, when you relax and so on.

The 'last straw' syndrome

Sometimes, if emotion is bottled up for a considerable amount of time, a valve blows and the person hits out – either literally or verbally. We have all experienced the problem of storing up anger and taking it out on someone else: a process that is sometimes called 'displacement'. The original object of our anger is now replaced by something or someone else. Again, the talking through of difficulties or the release of pent-up emotion can often help to ensure that the person does not feel the need to 'explode' in this way.

POSITIVE WAYS OF COPING WITH EMOTIONS

So far, we have discussed only the negative ways of dealing with emotion. Heron (1989a) identifies what he calls six 'positive' emotional states. These are: identification, acceptance, control, redirection, switching and transmutation. An understanding of the six can help in a broader understanding of how we may cope with emotional stress.

Identification

In this case, the person is aware of his or her emotional status. Stop reading for a moment and consider your *own* emotional status. Do you *know* what you are feeling at the moment or do you have to search around for words to describe what you are feeling? The person who can identify his or her feelings can experience them, own then and accept them as part of the human condition. It is possible to become increasingly aware of your emotional status merely by *choosing* to notice that status.

Acceptance

Once identification of emotions has occurred, the next step is to *accept* them. The temptation (particularly when the emotions are negative) is for us to want our emotions to be other than they are. We often chide ourselves for feeling a certain way. It could be otherwise. We could, usefully, *accept* what we are feeling and thus take further responsibility for ourselves and for our emotions.

Control

We cannot always express our feelings as we experience them. The health professional, for example, who always cries when a client starts crying, is unlikely to be able to support such clients for long: the whole process will become too emotionally exhausting. Instead, we can choose to *control* our feelings. That is not to say that we have to bottle them up indefinitely or repress them. It is to acknowledge that we can *choose* when we express them. The important point here, of course, is that we choose to express them *at some time*! The person who does not have positive emotional status often *believes* that he or she will discharge emotion at a later date but instead, bottles that emotion up or rationalizes it in one of the ways suggested above. The skill in controlling emotion lies also in being able to discharge it later.

Redirection

Sometimes we cannot express emotion directly. We may, for example, be unaware of the cause of our emotional state. Or we may have angry feelings that we cannot express directly towards a person (a dead relative, for example). In these cases we can choose to redirect our emotion through another channel: artistic expression, creative work or vigorous competitive exercise. Thus the emotion is released in a harmless and yet gratifying way.

Switching

It is tempting to believe that our emotions have control over us. We sometimes prefer to believe that we cannot choose our emotions. Another point of view is that we can acknowledge and accept our own feelings and, if we so choose, *switch* those feelings to others. For example, we may acknowledge that we are angry and unsettled and accept that. We may then consciously switch from an angry unsettled state to a more placid one, having made a contract with ourselves to return to explore the angry state at a later date. Again, the emphasis is on making sure that we *do* return to explore the anger.

This switching of emotions takes time and skill. We first need to be able to identify and accept our feelings. Once we have done that we are nearer to being able to make the mental adjustment required to shift a gear into a different and more positive state. Such emotional switching is of considerable importance to health professionals who constantly work with emotionally distressed clients. In a way, many health professionals already practice switching without really thinking about it. The point is to make the practice a *conscious* one.

Transmutation

In transmutation, the emotion is not merely switched nor is it redirected. Instead it is changed by the person through an internal process that allows the emotion to seep away and to become something more positive. Meditation and prayer are both examples of how strong negative emotions can be subtly transmuted into more serene ones. Being able to 'step outside' the emotion and being able to put it into a larger perspective can help too. For example, it is sometimes possible to identify a negative feeling and then to reflect on the status of that emotion in terms of one's entire life, or in terms of the entire world, or in terms of the whole history of the world: suddenly the steam is taken out of the emotion and it can very quickly evaporate into laughter or bemusement at ever having invested so much energy into what turns out to me a small matter.

These are processes for dealing with emotions positively. Sometimes emotions *cannot* be dealt with in this way: they need expression. In the next section, methods are described to help the release of bottled-up emotion. They are best used by people in pairs: one person has the bottled-up emotion, the other is a colleague or friend who is prepared to help. Having said that, many of these methods can be adapted for use by the person working alone. Once experience and familiarity have been gained in working with emotions in this way, and once the person has become skilled in the *positive* use of emotion, as described above, that person can continue to take charge of his or her own emotional status. The health professional who can identify, accept, express and redirect or transmute emotions in this way is increasing his or her emotional competence, is developing powerful ways of coping with stress and is also more likely to be effective in helping clients to deal with their own emotional needs and wants. One thing seems certain: we are unlikely to be able to help other people in their emotional upsets if we are unable to deal with our own feelings.

RELEASING BOTTLED-UP EMOTIONS

The techniques described here can be used by people in pairs though, as we noted above, some can be adapted for use by one individual. Once the particular technique has been learned through usage with a colleague or friend, it is often quite possible to use it on yourself. Clearly, these techniques should only be used when both parties have agreed to help each other. People should be forced into emotional disclosure if that is not something they would choose for themselves.

Literal description

Sometimes, when we are talking, we refer briefly to past events that may have been emotional. With this technique, the person is invited to return to that scene and describe it in detail. For example, a female social worker, in talking about her stress, suggests that:

... it used to be like this before ... I always used to get tense at home.

Her colleague suggests that she describes the past home situation in some detail:

... Well, it's not easy ... we lived in a terraced house ... our family spent a lot of time in the front room, around the TV.

Can you describe that room?

... It was fairly small ... my mother used to sit in a big armchair ... always in the same place.

27

As she describes the situation in close and literal detail, the emotions that are just beneath the surface emerge and she begins to cry. It seems that we are able to return to past events and when we describe them in detail we can often 'relive' the situation and express some of the pent-up emotion that was stored with the memory.

Present tense account

This is a variation on the above technique. Here, the colleague invites the social worker to describe the house that she lived in *the present tense*. Thus:

> . . . the front room is small . . . there is a TV in one corner . . . my mother's chair is over to one side and there is a large settee across one side of the room . . . there is a fireplace but we never have a fire in it.

This present tense account also takes the person back to an emotionally charged situation and allows her to explore it further and to experience, once again, the feelings she had at that time.

Early remembrances of a feeling

This is helpful in identifying feelings from the past that affect the way we feel in the present. In this example, Jane, a nurse, is talking about her feelings to a colleague:

> I'm finding it hard going at the moment. I've been on the same ward for over six months now and I'm bored.
>
> *Can you remember a time when you felt bored like this before?*
>
> Yes! When I was at school! . . . I used to sit and want the class to be over . . . I used to get angry that I had to sit there. Then I just gave up and resigned myself to the fact that I had to be there.
>
> *What are you feeling now?*
>
> Angry! I'm angry that I've been stuck on this ward for so long! I'm going to *do* something about it!

Here, the realization that the boredom had been experienced before and that it involved the bottling up of anger, led to a clearer appreciation of the *underlying* feeling. In this example, the realization led to an undertaking to take action to change the situation. Notice that the colleague asks 'What are you feeling now?' This is a useful check when any of these techniques are being used. It helps the other person to identify *present time* feelings, to acknowledge those feelings and to own them.

Contradiction

Sometimes we say exactly the opposite of what we mean. In this example, a physiotherapy student is talking about his feelings about his training.

I enjoy the job. Its not the job that is bothering me . . . I don't know quite what it is but it isn't work.

Try saying the opposite of that.

It *is* the work! I *hate* the job!

What does that feel like?

There's something in it . . . the more I think about it, the more I realize that it *is* the job that is getting me down.

Giving permission

This simply involves the colleague 'allowing' the other person to express pent-up feelings. Sometimes we need to be told by another person that we may cry or get angry. Thus, the colleague may say:

You sound pretty upset . . . It's alright with me if you cry.

Locating and developing a feeling in terms of the body

Often, pent-up emotion gets trapped in the body's musculature. Sometimes we can feel tension in a particular part of the body. Exploring this feeling sometimes leads to the *expression* of that feeling. In this example, one female nurse is talking to another about work in a medical ward.

I get very tense when I'm under pressure. Its horrible, I get all knotted up . . .

Are you feeling like that now?

Yes, a bit . . .

Where are your feelings that knotting up . . . in terms of your body?

Here, in my stomach . . .

Can you increase that feeling?

Yes . . . (*begins to cry*).

This approach, in helping the person to focus on the physical manifestation of a feeling, allows for the exploration and expression of it.

Rehearsal

We often 'rehearse' what we want to say to other people, or *would* say to them if we had the courage. This technique is an extension of that as it encourages a person to put into words what they are thinking. For example:

I get so angry with him.

If you could say anything to him, what would you say?

I'd tell him to bugger off! (*laughs*)

How does that feel?

Well, I wouldn't really say that to him, but I think if I toned it down a bit I *could* tell him what I think of him.

These are a few techniques that can be used by one person to help another express bottled-up emotion. Used sensitively, they can help the other person to identify and make sense of a whole range of feelings that were previously submerged. Sometimes, just the acknowledgement of the feeling is sufficient to make the other person feel relief. At other times, the person needs to express the emotion in full. Thus, they may find themselves crying or laughing. The great temptation will always be for the other person to intervene and calm them down, or 'reassure' them. It is suggested that it may be more therapeutic to *allow* the other person to express the emotion in full and that such expression can help in the total process of dealing with stress. Instead of carrying a lot of pent-up emotion, the person, at last, finds the space to release it and thus becomes free to think differently about his or her situation. It seems that pent-up emotion often gets in the way of clear thinking.

After emotional release has occurred, people often begin to think things through differently. For this reason, it is useful if a colleague or friend simply sits with them and allows them to piece things together. No advice or prescription is necessary here: people who have expressed emotion usually have all they need within themselves to make sense of what has happened.

As we noted above, these techniques can also be used by a person working alone. In this case, the person consciously 'literally describes' a situation or locates a 'bodily' feeling body and increases that feeling. After the resulting feeling has been expressed, the person may want to sit quietly and notice the new ideas and perceptions that tend to flood the mind following emotional release. This ability to take control of emotional release is all part of the process of developing enhanced emotional competence. To be able to 'unbottle' emotions in this way can not only help a person to cope with stress, it can also increase that person's skills in coping with the stresses and emotions of others. All health professionals frequently deal with the feelings of others. It would seem reasonable to suggest that all health professionals can become more therapeutic by learning to cope with their own emotions as well as those of other people.

SUMMARY

The nature of the emotions has been explored and some of the ways in which we choose to avoid reality have been examined. This chapter has considered both negative and positive ways of dealing with emotions and has identified practical ways of enabling the health professional to express bottled-up emotion.

3

Stress and self-awareness

Sometimes, in the middle of all this, I lose sight of *my* needs and who I am . . .

Student nurse

Aims of this chapter

This chapter explores:

- The notion of self
- Self-awareness
- Ways of becoming self-aware.

THE NOTION OF SELF

If we are to manage stress within ourselves, we need to get to know ourselves better. All health professions need self-awareness. It is the basic prerequisite of all skilful caring. But why? This chapter explores some of the reasons why all health professionals need to develop self-awareness in order to enhance their caring and to reduce stress.

What does it mean to talk about 'the self'? Of what is the self composed? Where is it? Is it part of our physical make up? Is it something spiritual? Is it something separate to the body and if so, what is its *relationship* to the body? Questions like these have interested philosophers and theologians for centuries. These days psychologists tackle the problem.

The existential school of philosophy discussed the issue under the heading of 'ontology': the study of being. To talk of the self, for the existentialists, is to talk of something more than just bodily existence. It is to describe the fact of being a conscious, knowing human being. It must be noted, however, that an notion of 'self' must also clearly be rooted in a *physical* existence.

Stress in Health Care: a Case in Point 4

A relaxation group is set up in a physiotherapy department of a general hospital for the staff who work in that department. The group is held during the lunch hour, twice a week. A variety of relaxation scripts are used, read by one of the physiotherapists.

A number of the physiotherapists find that, paradoxically, they are feeling more tense after the relaxation sessions. After discussion, it is realized that two things are happening. First, the sessions are being held in a room in which many of the physiotherapists feel they will be interrupted during the session by people coming through the door. Second, because of inexperience, the leader rushes through the script and does not allow sufficient time, afterwards, for the group to appreciate feeling relaxed. As a result, the group sessions **increase** *rather than reduce tension. After the group has moved to another room and the leader has gained confidence in the method, members of the group begin to feel the benefit.*

Sartre (1956) has described the notion 'authenticity': the state of true and honest presentation of being. Sartre's novel *Nausea*, (1965) was a literary description of a man's struggle to live an authentic life. He was later to acknowledge that the novel was biographical (Sartre, 1964). The authentic person, for Sartre, was one who consistently acts in accordance with his or her own values, wishes and feelings, making no attempt to play act or to adopt a façade. That person also recognizes the 'being' of others and realizes that when he or she is with someone else, that other person is also a conscious, valuing, thinking being.

Sartre illustrates the opposite of authenticity well in a vignette. He describes a young boy and girl sitting at a café table. They are slowly developing a relationship. Tentatively, the boy puts out his hand and affectionately holds the girl's hand. The girl, not knowing how to respond, chooses to pretend that the while incident has not occurred and almost 'disowns' her own hand. She turns it into an object. It is as if her hand was merely an impersonal appendage. Perhaps, too, the boy turns the girl into an object by not appreciating the confusion he is causing and by not withdrawing his hand. This, for Sartre, is inauthenticity: the turning of ourselves, and others, into objects. Arguably, we do just this when we are under intense stress. We begin to treat ourselves as though we were objects rather than living, breathing, feeling subjects. When we return to being 'subjects', we can once again meet others as subjects.

Martin Buber (1958) calls the meeting of two 'subjects' the I–Thou relationship: the meeting of two people who respect each other's humanity. He contrasts the I–Thou relationship with the I–It relationship. The person who adopts an I–It stance in relationship with another person does not recognize the other as a human being (with all that involves) but treats the other as an 'object'. We can probably all recall times when, under stress, we have treated patients or clients as objects. Sometimes we label the 'It' an 'appendicectomy' or a 'case'. While, if we can allow ourselves a moment's thought, we know that underneath this label there are other persons with thoughts, feelings, families and all sorts of problems, and yet we can find no other way of coping with them at this particular moment other than by seeing them as clinical objects. Unfortunately, for some, this tendency to treat people as objects becomes a way of life: the patient or client remains more interesting as a clinical entity than as a person.

Arguably, health professionals who have become so alienated from their patients have also become alienated from themselves. Perhaps chronic, job-related stress causes this two-way alienation. The process of constantly caring for others can indeed be stressful.

R. D. Laing developed these notions and wrote of the 'true' and 'false' self (Laing, 1959). The true self is the inner, private sense of self. The false self is the outer, often pretending sense of self. According to Laing, the true self often watches what the false self is doing and a sense of contempt is experienced. The false self is often compliant to the demands of others and can be artificial and insincere. In Sartre's terms, the false self acts inauthentically. The person who has a strong sense of the true self and is able to act authentically and genuinely is deemed by Laing to have ontological security: security and strength of being. Such security can allow a person to feel able to act rather than to feel acted upon, to make decisions and to feel generally more autonomous. Such a person is also likely to respect the autonomy and self-respect of others. This is not to be confused with selfishness or arrogance – quite the opposite. The ontologically secure person is all too aware of human frailty yet, despite it, remains determined to act in a genuine and honest way. That takes courage.

We can see examples of Sartre's and Laing's ideas in health care practice. When I was a patient in hospital, I became very aware of how some nurses adopt the 'role of the nurse' as they enter a ward: they suddenly become 'someone else'. It is as though they leave part of themselves behind as they go to work. They have one 'self' for their patients and another for friends and colleagues. If we notice that we are 'acting the role of the health professional' in talking with patients, rather than being ourselves, then we are acting in an inauthentic manner. This is not a plea for lack of professionalism but just an observation that there is a world of difference between the health professional who is open, genuine and sincere and the one who adopts a professional façade, an artificial manner and who fools no one – neither self, colleagues nor least of all patients. The health professional who begins to develop self-awareness can monitor her behaviour and note tendencies towards adopting such a veneer. She can also reduce her stress levels by acting 'naturally'. Putting up a façade can be a stressful business.

PSYCHOLOGICAL VIEWS OF THE SELF

Psychologists have approached the concept of self from a variety of view points. Some have attempted to analyse the factors that go to make up the self rather in the way that a chemist might try to discover the chemicals that have gone to into a mixture. Others have argued that there are certain consistent aspects of the self that determine to some extent the way in which we conduct our lives. Psychoanalytical theory argues that early childhood experiences affect and shape the self, determining how, as adults, we react to the world about us. Childhood experiences lay foundations of the self which may be modified through the process of growing up but which, nevertheless, stay with us throughout our lives. Such a view is 'deterministic': our present sense of self is determined by earlier life experiences. We develop our present sense of self out of our past.

Other psychologists question such reductionist theories – theories that attempt to analyse the self into parts. Instead, they prefer to view the self from a holistic or gestalt perspective. The gestalt approach argues that the whole or totality of the self is always something different to, and larger than, the sum of the aspects that make it up. Just as we cannot discover the true nature of a piece of music by examining the piece note by note, neither can we understand the self, completely, by analysing it into separate aspects.

Still other psychologists take the view that the sense of self is dynamic and everchanging. There is no core or 'real' self. What we call 'self' at any given time is that moment's set of beliefs, values and ideas that colour our view of the world. George Kelly (1955) suggested the metaphor of 'goggles': we all look at the world, at ourselves and at others, through different goggles that are coloured by our beliefs, values and experiences up to that moment. As our beliefs, values and experiences change, so do the tints of our 'goggles'. Thus, for Kelly, the individual is in a constant state of flux – developing, growing and changing as life is encountered. For Kelly, we *are* what we perceive ourselves to be or, as the novelist Kurt Vonnegut put it: 'We are what we pretend to be' (Vonnegut, 1968). In addition Kelly noted that we *are* also what *other people* perceive us to be. In other words, we are not only 'selves' for us, but also 'selves' for other people.

We do not exist in isolation. What we are and who we are depends upon the other people with whom we live, work and relate. Our sense of self often depends upon the report about us that we receive from others. In this sense, other people are telling us who we are. As health care professionals we rely on patients, colleagues, educators and managers offering us both positive and negative feedback. We absorb such feedback and incorporate the bits that we need to into our sense of self. Sometimes reports from others seem important: at other times they seem less necessary.

ASPECTS OF THE SELF

The self, then, is a complicated concept. It is worth emphasizing the word *concept*. The self is not a *thing* in the way that our livers or lungs are 'things'. The notion of self is an abstraction, a way of talking. It is a shorthand for that part of us that is concerned with thinking, feeling, valuing, evaluating and so forth. While, in one sense, the mind and body are one, in another, they are different if only in that the mind is a *thing*, an object in the world, while the 'self' is a construct. To talk about 'mind and body' is tricky, for that suggests that two similar sorts of items are under discussion. One way of clarifying what is contained within the concept of self is to consider the notion of *personhood*. If we can identify those basic criteria that distinguish persons from other sorts of things we may be clearer about what it means to talk about the self. Bannister and Fransella (1986) maintain that such a list of criteria for personhood will include at least the following items. It is argued that you consider yourself a person in that you:

(a) entertain a notion of your own separateness from others: you rely on the privacy of your own consciousness;
(b) entertain a notion of the integrality of completeness of your experience, so that all parts of it are relatable because you are the experiencer;
(c) entertain a notion of your own continuity over time; you possess your own biography and live in relation to it;
(d) entertain a notion of the causality of your actions; you have purposes, you intend, you accept a partial responsibility for the effects of what you do;
(e) entertain a notion of other persons by analogy with yourself; you assume a comparability of subjective experience.

These criteria bring together many of the ideas discussed above. They acknowledge the person's uniqueness and difference to others; they acknowledge the person's continuity with the past and the acknowledge a relatedness with other people. We do not exist in isolation: we can assume that we share the planet with other people who are, to a greater or lesser degree, like us. We can assume, also, that those other people, like ourselves, experience degrees of stress. If we can learn to understand our own stress and stressors, we may be in a better position to understand the stresses of others. A simple way of acknowledging the fact that we are unique in some respects but, in other respects, are like others, is via the following triplet attributed to the psychologist Gordon Allport. All persons are in some ways:

– like *no* other persons;
– like *some* other persons;
– like *all* other persons.

Another way of considering the concept of self is to consider *aspects* of it. While, as we have noted, all the aspects tend to work together (we hope!) in harmony, they are most easily discussed as parts. John Rowan has taken almost a similar approach in his discussion of 'subpersonalities' (Rowan, 1989), which he describes as semi-permanent, semi-autonomous regions of the personality. The analysis offered here is not an exhaustive one of all aspects of the self (as we noted above, what *individuals* call 'self' will vary from person to person); it is offered as a means of highlighting the complex and multi-faceted nature of the concept of self. The aspects of self discussed here are:

- The physical aspect
- The spiritual aspect
- The darker aspect
- The social aspect.

The physical aspect of self

The physical aspect of the self is the bodily, 'felt' sense of self: it includes the totality of our physical bodies. One way of considering the self, in fact, is to consider that sense as being a product of the body: bodies generate 'selves'. After all, the chemistry that goes to make up our bodies is also the chemistry that produces our 'mind', which in turn, produces our sense of self. The physical aspect of self covers all those things such as how we feel about our bodies, our sense of body image, our appreciation of how fat or thin we are and so on. It is notable (rather painfully, sometimes) that *our own* perception of our body is not necessarily the perception that others have. It is notable, too, that the body often *tells* us that we are stressed. Our first indication of stress is often through muscle tension, uncomfortable feelings in the stomach or other psychosomatic indicators.

This physical sense of self can be put to the test now. Stop reading for a moment and check your own physical status. What do you notice, for instance, about your muscles: are they tense or relaxed? Notice the way that you are holding this book. Notice, too, the muscles in your shoulders. Hunched and tense shoulder muscles are often a sign of stress.

The spiritual aspect of self

Human beings seem to have an inbuilt need to invest what they do with meaning. The spiritual dimension of the person can be described as that part that is concerned with the development of personal meaning. For some, that sense of meaning will be framed in religious terms, but it may not be. For others, meaning may be discovered through philosophy, politics, psychology, sociology and so on. People's meaning systems vary both in their overall structure and in their content. One thing seems certain: it is meaning (or the search for it) that motivates us for much of the time. Jung (1938) described this question for meaning as 'individuation': the search for the self which was both lonely and difficult. He suggested that one possible outcome of individuation was the realization of both the individual nature of the person and also the person's unity with all other persons. In this context, Carl Rogers noted that 'what is most personal is most general' (Rogers, 1967): there is a certain universality about the business of being human. This notion of the spiritual or 'meaning' dimension of the self is explored further in Chapter 5. Under extreme stress we can question all sorts of aspects of meaning.

Practical Methods of Coping with Stress in the Health Professions: 3

A GIFT OF TIME

Most health professionals find that their schedule is inter-rupted at certain times. Appointments are cancelled or trav-elling makes time-keeping difficult. Next time you find that your schedule is disturbed and there is nothing you can do about it, allow yourself the Gift of Time. Rather than becoming increasingly more stressed because you are not doing what you planned to do, use the time you have constructively. Use it to plan ahead, to consider your own wishes and plans or, perhaps, to notice what is going on around you.

The darker aspect of self

There is an aspect in all of us that tends towards the negative. While it has become popular to discuss the positive aspects of

39

the self and to theorize about Maslow's (1972) notion of self-actualization – the realization of our full potential – there seems little doubt that we also have a darker side. Jung (1938) described this darker side as 'the shadow' and wrote about it thus:

> Unfortunately there is no doubt that man is, as a whole, less good than he imagines himself or wants to be. Everyone carries a shadow, and the less it is embodied in the individual's conscious life, the blacker and denser it is. . . .

Jung suggests that if we want truly to become self-aware, we must be prepared to explore that darker side of our personalities. No easy task! Most of us would rather deny that side of ourselves or rationalize our negative thoughts and behaviour. Sometimes, however, we give ourselves away: particularly through the use of the mental mechanism known as 'projection'. With projection we label others with qualities that are our own but of which we are unaware. Often we notice the bad bits of other people while studiously avoiding our own bad bits. This is very evident when we begin to get judgemental and pious about others. While 'the shadow' may not be the easiest aspect of ourselves to face, it is likely that acknowledging the darker side can help us to accept the darker side of others. It is often the darker side of ourselves that causes us the most internal stress. Perhaps if we can face and accept some of the darker aspects of our make up we can learn to live more easily with ourselves. We all tend to put a lot of energy into fighting those more negative aspects of ourselves. Unfortunately, too, when we are very stressed we can often find few resources to cope with the darker side of ourselves. It is at such time that we develop cynicism and perhaps a 'gallows' sense of humour. Perhaps such humour is one more way of coping with the unbearable.

Take some time to consider *your* darker side. How does the prospect feel to you? Do you dismiss the idea altogether as somehow too morbid? Do you acknowledge, readily, that the darker side is a side of you that you prefer to ignore? Or does the prospect of looking at your darker side make you anxious? In the end, Jung was optimistic about the person who faces the darker side. He was of the view that once people did this, they could then come to terms with many things about themselves. It seems that if we can face the more negative aspects of ourselves and accept them, then we can face most things.

The social aspect of self

The social self is that aspect of the person which is shared with others. It is our presentation of self in various social situations. Consider, for example, yourself at work. Consider, then, yourself at home. Finally, consider yourself with your closest friend. You may well find that you are considering almost three different people! We tend to modify aspects of our presentation of self according to the people we are with and according to what we anticipate will be their expectations of us. This social self, then, is closely linked to the self-as-defined-by-others. We do not live as isolated beings. We are dependent upon others to tell us about ourselves. More than that, we *are* different to different people. Consider how the following people view you: your mother, your teacher, your boy- or girlfriend or your partner. In each case, those people will see a different 'you' and yet they are all looking at the same person. When they look at you, what do they see? The person that *you* imagine yourself to be or someone quite different?

Consider, also, how *continuous* or otherwise your relationships with others are. Are you always 'the same' with other people? Do you sometimes find other people hard to bear? Are you constant with some people and changeable with others? Learning to notice how our relationships wax and wane is one more method of coping with stress – for other people can be as much a source of stress to us as we can be to ourselves. Sartre (1944) had a particularly bleak view of our relationships with others. In his play, *In Camera*, one of his characters declares that Hell is not some place opposite to Heaven but instead that 'Hell – it's other people'.

A MODEL OF THE SELF

These, then, are aspects of the self – a few aspects among many. What is required now is a model that helps to bring all of these aspects into perspective. In its simplest form, the self as a totality can be seen as being made up of three areas or focuses of interest. The model offered here (Fig. 3.1) is divided into two parts. The outer public aspect of the self is what others see of us. The inner public aspect is what goes on in our heads and bodies. In one way, the outer experience is what other people are most familiar

OUTER EXPERIENCE OF SELF	INNER EXPERIENCE OF SELF
• Movement • Speech • Eye Contact • Touch • Proximity to others • Gestures • Facial Expression	• Thinking • Feeling • Sensing • Intuiting • Bodily sensation

Figure 3.1 A model of the self.

with. We communicate the inner experience through the outer. Our thoughts and feelings are all communicated through this outer presentation of self. Of what does it consist?

THE OUTER EXPERIENCE OF THE SELF

At the most obvious, behaviour consists of body movements: the turning of the head, the crossing of arms and legs, hand movements, walking, running and so on. At a more subtle level the issue becomes more involved. We can note a great variety of less obvious behaviours that convey something about the inner sense of self.

First is speech. Clearly, what we say and the words and phrases we use are a potent means by which we convey thoughts and feelings to others. Why we choose *these* particular words and phrases, however, depends on our past experiences, our education, our social position, our attitudes, values and beliefs and on the company that we are in when we use those words. Often, too, we talk using a particular set of personal 'catchphrases' and sayings that are peculiar to us. Indeed, we are often recognized by them. Running alongside speech are the non-linguistic aspects of speech: timing, pacing, volume, minimal prompts (mm's and yes's), the use of silence and so on. The use of such non-linguistic aspects of speech can be a powerful way of conveying our inner selves to others. As we noted above, we are always communicating – even when we think we are not!

When we talk to others we invariably look at them (although this aspect of communication is culture-specific: not all people in all cultures engage in eye contact when they talk to each other). As Heron (1970a) notes, there can be a wide variety in the intensity, amount and quality of eye contact. When we are embarrassed or upset, for example, we make less eye contact. When we are emotionally close to another person, our eye contact is often sustained. We can learn to become conscious of our use of what must be the most powerful aspect of communication and to monitor the amount and quality of our eye contact. We should also remain aware of the *cultural* differences that are involved here. People from cultures very different to our own use eye contact in other ways. It is important that we do not interpret such different use of eye contact inappropriately. It is also important that we respect the differences in use of eye contact from one person (of one culture) to another.

It is interesting to note what happens to our eye contact when we are stressed. As a general rule, it is probably true that we find direct eye contact with others difficult when we are under stress. Next time you are stressed, pay attention to your eye contact and note the degree to which you find it difficult. Then ask yourself 'What is *making* it difficult?' You can gain considerable self-insight in the process.

Touch, in relation to others, is another important aspect of our outer experience. Typically, in this culture, we touch more those people to whom we are close: members of the family, lovers and very close friends. Health care involves a high degree of this personal aspect of human interaction and it is important that, as with eye contact, we learn to monitor and consciously use the facility of touch. It is worth noting, too, that some people are 'frequent touchers' and others 'infrequent touchers'. Some people like being touched and like touching others: other people are repelled by it. Also, all touching should be unambiguous: clearly, touch has sexual connotations for some people. Touch also has a direct bearing on the relief of stress. Stress often manifests itself in the form of muscular tension. Such tension can often be reduced through massage. Bond (1986) offers a number of simple approaches to the issue of how to offer massage to another person.

When we communicate verbally with others, we tend to stand or sit close to them. How near we stand or sit in relation to others is determined by a number of factors – the level of intimacy we have with them, our relationship with them and whether or not we are dominant or submissive in that relationship (Brown, 1965). In the health care professions, carers tend to be in a dominant position *vis-à-vis* their patients and will tend to stand closer to their patients than would be the case in ordinary day-to-day relationships. It is useful to imagine that we are surrounded by an invisible bubble, the threshold of which can only be crossed by certain other people. If people accidentally break through the bubble and touch us, they tend to withdraw quickly to avoid embarrassment to both parties.

The issue of proximity to others needs close consideration. We need to become aware of how close or distant we like to be in relation to others. We need also to note other people's preferences and to be sensitive towards them. One useful way of judging this distance between you and the other person is to allow the other person to set that distance. In other words, you invite the other person to draw up a chair or you allow that person to determine where *he* or *she* will stand in relation to you, and not vice versa. Once again, as we become more self-aware, we gain more insight into the needs and wants of others. Notice, too, how stressful too close a proximity can be.

One of the clearest indicators of our inner experience is facial expression. Frowns and smiles do much to convey the feelings that are being experienced inside. It is important that facial expression and speech are congruent or matched. We have all experienced people who *say* that they are cheerful or upset, but whose facial expressions suggest otherwise. Bandler and Grinder (1975) note that, for the purposes of clear communication, three aspects of our outer behaviour must match: general body position, content of speech and facial expression. If two or more of these are mismatched then our communication will be confused and confusing. Thus if we *say* that we are cheerful but shrug our shoulders and have an unhappy expression, the message will be unclear. We can do a lot to improve our communication on this level. It is insufficient just to *say* what we mean; we must also be *seen* to mean it.

Stress also shows itself in the facial expression. Frowning, a tightness around the mouth and eyes are all characteristic of someone who is stressed. Sometimes, the process of consciously allowing those muscle clusters to relax can bring about a degree of relief from physical tension associated with stress.

Two issues become clear from this brief analysis of the outer aspects of self. We can become aware of our use of speech, eye contact, touch, proximity to others, gesture, facial expression and non-linguistic aspects of speech as a means of deepening our understanding of ourselves. Also, by becoming conscious of how we use those verbal and non-verbal behaviours we can use them more skilfully to enhance our contact with others. We can increase our interpersonal skills by intentionally using ourselves as instruments. Heron (1973) uses the expression 'conscious use of self' to convey this concept. This is not to say that we need to become robotic and artificial but to note that in caring for others we can more precisely use our 'selves' as instruments of communication. We also need to be able to communicate our inner feelings with ourselves. This may sound odd but many people emotionally 'freeze' when they are under stress. To remain in contact with what is going on inside is an important strategy in dealing with the consequences of stress. That inner aspect of the self is now examined in more detail.

THE INNER EXPERIENCE OF THE SELF

The inner, private experience in this model (Fig. 3.1) may be divided into four aspects of mental functioning – thinking, feeling, sensing and intuiting – and the experience of the body. Clearly, the division of these aspects into two groups is artificial as both mental and physical events are interrelated. As Searle (1983) points out, a mental event is also a physical event. To think that it is not is to perpetuate the old philosophical problem of mind/body dualism. This is sometimes known as Cartesian dualism after the philosopher Rene Descartes, who believed that mental and physical events could be considered separately. Today, the tendency is towards healing this split and interest continues to develop in concepts of holistic health care and holistic medicine – both of which treat the mind and body together. As we have already noted, any concept of the self must take into account the mind and the body as a totality.

The thinking dimension

In this model, thinking refers to all the aspects, logical and otherwise, of our mental processes. One moment's reflection on thinking will reveal that it is not a linear process. We do not think in sentences or even in the series of phrases. The process is much more haphazard than that. The technique known as 'free association', used in psychoanalysis, demonstrates the apparently random nature of some of our thinking. Free association demands that the individual verbalizes whatever comes into the mind, with no attempt to censor or stop the flow. Try to do this. The process is always difficult and sometimes impossible. The reasons for this are outlined in the psychoanalytical literature and such theory can offer insights into the genesis and nature of thought processes. Clearly, not everyone wants or can afford psychoanalysis, but its ideas can be useful in attempting to understand thinking.

Arguably, the domain of thinking is more dominant in certain individuals. Certainly, thinking is highly rated in our culture and the education system sometimes seems to concern itself *only* with this mode. The domains of feeling, sensing and intuiting are usually less well catered for. In health care, however, we are concerned with all sorts of feelings, from pain to anxiety, from depression to elation. Understanding these requires the use of dimensions other than thinking. On the other hand, it is obviously important that we all develop the thinking aspect. If we are to progress as a research-based profession and if we are to be able to demonstrate critical awareness, we must be able to think clearly. We must also be able to appreciate when feeling obstructs thinking, and vice versa.

The feeling dimension

Feeling in this model refers to the emotional aspect of the person: love, sadness, joy, happiness, etc. Heron (1977) argues that four dominant aspects of emotion are frequently denied and repressed in our culture: anger, grief, fear and embarrassment. He argues that anger can be expressed through loud sound and shouting, grief through tears, fear through trembling and embarrassment through laughter. He argues, further, that such expression of emotion (or catharsis) is a healthy process. Heron claims that we live in a non-cathartic culture and the general tendency is to encourage people to control rather than to express emotion. As a result, we all carry a pool of unexpressed emotion which distorts our thinking and stops us functioning fully. If we can learn to express some of this bottled-up emotion, and methods of doing this will be discussed later, then we can become more open to experience, less fearful and anxious and can exercise more self-determination and autonomy. Part of becoming self-aware entails discovering and exploring the emotional dimension.

Health care professionals must deal with other people's emotions and there is a link between the way in which we handle our own emotions and the way in which we handle the emotions of others. If we understand and can express our own anger, frustration, fear, grief and embarrassment, we shall be better able to handle those emotions in other people. In caring for others, we must get to know ourselves better. We can also learn to handle our own stress through knowing ourselves better. We may not be able to change all the outside stressors but we can certainly monitor our own reactions to those stressors. Once identified, those reactions can be monitored.

Certainly other people's emotions affect us and stir up our own, unexpressed emotions. Try this simple experiment. Next time a programme on television moves you near to tears, turn off the set and allow yourself to cry. As you do so, reflect on what it is you are crying about. It is highly likely that the issue causing the tears is personal, and is not directly related to the television programme. Most people carry this unexpressed emotion just beneath the surface. Health care professionals who work in particularly emotionally charged environments – children's wards, intensive therapy units, psychiatric units and so forth – may want to consider self-help methods for exploring their own hidden emotions. Co-counselling, discussed in the next chapter, is one such method and others are discussed by Bond (1986) and Bond and Kilty (1983). Alternatively, consider going to the cinema as a means of emotional release. Why do most people go to the cinema? To cry, to allow themselves to be frightened or to laugh. The cinema and, to a lesser extent, the theatre, concerts and sporting events offer 'natural' release valves for people's pent-up emotion.

The sensing dimension

The sensing dimension in the model refers to inputs through the five special senses: touch, taste, smell, hearing, sight and also to proprioceptive and kinaesthetic senses. Proprioception refers to our ability to know the position of our bodies and thus to know where we are in space. We do not, for instance, need to *think* about our body position most of the time. We are fed that information by bundles of nerve fibres known as proprioceptors. Kinaesthetic sense refers to our sense of body movement. Again, this is not a sense that we normally have to think about.

We can make ourselves aware of any of the senses. Another simple experiment will demonstrate this. Stop reading for a moment and pay attention to everything that you can hear. Take in all the sounds around you: the more subtle as well as the more obvious. In doing so, notice how much of this particular sense is normally ignored and how many sounds are usually filtered out of consciousness. At times it is vital that our senses are selective and that extraneous sounds, images, smells and so on are banished from awareness. On the other hand, that filtering mechanism often becomes *too* efficient and we filter out or fail to notice many sounds and sights that are around us all the time. We live half asleep.

In developing an awareness of our senses, we can begin to notice the world again. Just as importantly, we can begin to notice *each other* again. In developing our sense of sight, for instance, we can begin to notice subtle changes in other people's expressions, body postures and other aspects of non-verbal communication. Without that awareness we may miss a considerable amount of essential interpersonal information. In health care, the value of such awareness is clear. Health care professionals need to be observant. What is not always so clear is *how* health care professionals are supposed to become observant. Like any other skill development, training to notice takes time and practice. The redeeming feature is that it is a skill which each *individual* can develop. In a way, it is simply a matter of **remembering** to notice. Eventually, such awareness or 'staying awake' becomes part of the person.

The intuitive dimension

The intuitive dimension is perhaps the most undervalued. Intuition refers to knowledge and insight that arrives independently of the senses. In other words we just 'know'. Ornstein (1975), who studied the literature on the differences between the two sides of the brain, identified intuition with the right side. He argued that the two sides have qualitatively different functions: the left side is concerned with cognitive processes and with rationality; the right is more to do with holism, creativity and intuition.

If he is right, the implication is that if the intuitive aspect is developed further (along with creativity) then both sides of the brain will function optimally. Ornstein argues that the present Western culture is dominated by the left brain approach to education and development. He calls for an educational system that honours creativity and intuition *alongside* the development of rationality.

Perhaps we neglect intuition through fear of it or concern that it may not be trusted. On the other hand, it is likely that we all have 'hunches' that when followed turn out to be 'right'. Many aspects of nursing require the health care professional to be intuitive. Sometimes, in order to empathize with another person, we have to guess what they are feeling. Sometimes we seem to 'know' what they are feeling. Certainly, group work and counselling depend to a fair degree on this intuitive ability. Carl Rogers, founder of client-centred counselling, noted that when he had a hunch about something that was happening in a counselling session, it invariably helped if he verbalized that intuition (Rogers, 1967). Using intuition consciously and openly takes courage and sometimes it is wrong. On the other hand, used hand-in-hand with more traditional forms of thinking, it can enhance the health care professional/patient relationship in a way that logic, on its own, never can.

The experience of the body

The fifth aspect of the model of self-awareness is the experience of the body. If the mind and body are directly interrelated, in fact inseparable, then any mental activity will affect the body, and vice versa. It is notable, however, that much of the literature in health care and medicine divides the person up into separate psychological entities. Indeed, the two spheres are treated, typically, by different practitioners: general health care professionals care for physical ailments and psychiatric health care professionals deal with psychological problems.

It is easy to talk as though the mind and body *were* separate. Indeed, we do not *have* a mind/body, we *are* our mind/body. Everything that we refer to as being part of our mind and body is part of ourselves. Expressions such as 'I'm not happy with my body . . .' or 'I've got that sort of mind . . .' indicate how easy it is for us to dissociate ourselves from either the body or the mind.

Perhaps, when we are under stress, it is easier for us to live in this way. It is rather as if we stop listening to what our body is telling us: usually, to slow down!

Coming to notice body feelings takes times and patience. Of course, appreciation of inner bodily experiences are limited to some degree by the supply of sensory nerve endings to certain aspects of the body. Some parts are better served than others. On the other hand, it is easy to lose touch with those bodily sensations of which we *may* become aware. Before you read any further, just take a moment to notice what is going on inside your body. What do you notice? Are there areas of muscle tension? Are the muscles of your stomach pulled in tightly? Can you become aware of your breathing? Are you breathing deeply into your stomach or is your breathing light and shallow? What happens when you make small changes to your body? What happens when you relax sets of muscles or change your breathing?

All the information that can be gleaned from the body can enable us to appreciate something about our psychological status. Tension in sets of muscles, for example, may be the first we know of the fact that we are anxious or tense. Learning to 'listen' to the body in this way can help us to more accurately assess our true feelings about ourselves and others. Wilhelm Reich (1949), a psychoanalyst who was particularly interested in the mind/body relationship, advanced the notion of 'character armour'. Reich maintained that our emotional feelings could become trapped within sets of muscles and consequently affect posture and movement. He suggested that direct manipulation of those sets of muscles could release the emotion trapped within them with characteristic emotional release of catharsis. Such work on the body has become known as Reichian bodywork (Totton and Edmonston, 1988) and can be a powerful and effective means of developing self-awareness through direct body contact. These measures can also be effective in reducing stress levels.

Similar but different methods of this sort which involve direct physical contact include Rolfing (Rolf, 1973), bioenergetics (Lowen, 1967) and Feldenkrais (Feldenkrais, 1972), three bodywork methods that have developed out of Reich's original formulation. Again, these methods offer very positive and physical ways of tackling the problem of stress that manifests itself through physical tension.

Less dramatic but valid methods of body/mind exploration include: massage, yoga, the martial arts, certain types of meditation, the Alexander technique (Alexander, 1969), dance and certain types of sport. Examples of meditation techniques are included in Chapter 6 of this book.

All these methods can enhance awareness of self through attention to changes in the body and thus create insight into psychological states. They can also aid the development of awareness of body image. Observations of people in everyday life will reveal how frequently people walk around with lop-sided shoulders, a stooping gait or even with each side of their face showing different expressions. Often, too, they seem to be totally unaware of these things. Bodywork methods can enable the individual to develop greater physical symmetry and balance, better posture, improved breathing and a healthier physical status, generally. All aspects of health care call for psychological and physical stamina and are taxing on the mind/body. These methods in combination with more traditional approaches to self-awareness can lead to a powerful and healthy approach to self-care. Perhaps burnout, so frequently a problem of occupations that depend upon a high degree of human contact, can be prevented effectively through this mix of attention to the body and mind.

SELF-AWARENESS

A model of the self has been outlined which takes account of the inner and outer aspects of the concept and which has attempted to marry the mind and body. The question now arises: 'What is self-awareness?'

A first point that needs to be made is that what is *not* being discussed is 'self-consciousness', in the everyday sense of the word. To be self-conscious is to be embarrassed by ourselves, to be painfully aware of our being observed by others. Sartre (1956) describes this well when he suggests that under the scrutinizing gaze of the other person, we are turned into an object, a 'thing'. It is our response to being treated in this way that causes us to become self-conscious. For the very self-conscious person, he or she can exaggerate this sense of being treated as an object. In being too acutely aware of other people's attention, the person imagines the scrutiny to be more acute than is actually the case. It is rather like having someone watch us undertaking a skill such as giving an injection. We tend to become deskilled by their watching and imagine they are being highly critical. Self-consciousness is a bit like this. It tends to make you awkward and to make you feel criticized. This is true, for example, of the adolescents who imagine (usually falsely) that they are being observed through highly critical eyes. Their own sense of insecurity is projected onto the world and they imagine that others view them as harshly and as critically as they view themselves.

Clearly, such self-consciousness is more of a hindrance than a help when it comes to relating to others, as any acutely shy person knows. Yet such self-consciousness is far removed from self-awareness and may indicate a false or exaggerated self-concept.

Self-awareness refers to the gradual and continuous process of noticing and exploring aspects of the self, whether behavioural, psychological or physical, with the intention of developing personal and interpersonal understanding. Such awareness is probably best not developed for its own sake: it is intimately bound up with our relationships with others. To become more aware, and to have a deeper understanding of ourselves is to have a sharper and clearer picture of what is happening to others. In this sense, it is a process of discrimination. The more that we can discriminate ourselves from others, the more we can understand our similarities. If we are unaware and blind to ourselves, then we are likely to remain blind to others. A rather crude illustration may help to drive this point home. If I buy a bright green sweater, I immediately notice how many other people are wearing bright green sweaters – a fact of which I was not aware before the purchase. In noticing that fact about others I can also notice other things about them. And so, if I let it, the process escalates. I can notice not only the subtle differences between persons but also their similarities. The point to note is that the process begins with me. I must first examine myself.

Such a process of examination requires patience and honesty. It is easy to fall into the trap of *interpreting* thoughts, feelings and behaviour, rather than (initially at least) merely noticing them. That interpretation logically comes *after* we have gathered the data, after we have clearly described to ourselves our present status. This stage of self-awareness training may be likened to the assessment stage of the health care process. Information about the self is gathered in order to develop a clearer picture before any attempt is made to solve problems, decide upon changes, or identify reasons for the way we are.

This approach may be described as phenomenological (Spinelli, 1989). Phenomenology is a branch of philosophy that is concerned with attempting to *describe* things as they appear to be without recourse to making value-judgements about them. Thus, in the human context, a phenomenological approach to self-awareness training would concern itself purely with *describing* aspects of the self as they surface and become known. Such an approach demands that we suspend judgement on ourselves. Instead of telling ourselves that 'this bit of me is OK . . . this bit is bad and needs to be changed', we merely note that *it is as it is*. Once we have more data at our disposal, the answer to the question 'why?' may become self-evident. If we jump to hasty conclusions we may either be harshly critical of ourselves or wreck the project altogether because we are disenchanted. Certainly, the road to self-awareness is not an easy one to tread, but the phenomenological approach can make it bearable. After all, if *we* do not accept ourselves, who will? If we do not accept ourselves, shall we accept other people? One of the first things we have to do when trying to cope with stress is to accept the fact that we *are* stressed.

This method of description rather than interpretation is of great value in group settings and in counselling. Thus it may be used to help other individuals and groups of individuals to work out coping strategies. In this role, the facilitator of the group does not attempt to offer interpretations of what is happening in the group, but limits his or her role to descriptions of events and of behaviours and encourages other group members to do the same. In the context of counselling, the phenomenological approach also pays dividends. If we can stand back and avoid interpreting what it is we think our clients are saying, we give them the chance to make *their own* interpretations. This attitude towards counselling is known as the client-centred approach (Rogers, 1967; Burnard, 1989). It is argued that the only individual who *can* make a valid interpretation of a person's behaviour is that person. If other people are to be helped with their stress, it is important that we do not, too readily, become *prescriptive*.

DEVELOPING SELF-AWARENESS

There are various ways of developing self-awareness. Some involve introspection and some entail involvement with and feedback from other people. Any course leading towards self-awareness must contain both facets: the inner search and the observations of others. Introspection by itself can lead to a one-sided, totally subjective view of the self. It is difficult, if not impossible, for people working alone to transcend themselves and take the larger view. In order to balance that subjective view, we need the view of others.

Before examining some of the methods of introspection and group work, it is useful to note one simple method of enhancing self-awareness: the process of noticing what we are doing, the process of self-monitoring. All that this involves is that you remain conscious of what you are doing as you do it. In other words, you 'stay awake' and develop the skill of keeping your attention focused on your actions, both verbal and non-verbal. Such a process, while easy in theory, can be quite difficult in practice. It is easy to become distracted by inner thoughts and preoccupations so that our actions become automatic and unnoticed – even robotic.

Awareness of our focus of attention has implications for all aspects of health care. The health care professionals who are able to keep their attention focused out for longer periods is likely to become more observant and more accurate in those observations. The health care professionals who can differentiate between what they are thinking and feeling 'inside' and what is going on 'outside' are less likely to jump to conclusions about observations or to make value judgements based on prejudice rather than on fact. They are also likely to be more effective as critical thinkers and more able to assess and evaluate new ideas and new theories.

All such explorations can be carried out either in isolation, with another person or in groups. To explore the self in the company of another person can be a rewarding and economical method. Economical in that the time available can be equally divided between the two people. Co-counselling offers a useful format for such exploration, and this is explained in Chapter 8.

Other methods of self-awareness training include the use of role-play, social skills training, meditation and assertiveness skills training. These methods are well documented in the literature (see, for example, Kagan, 1985; Hargie et al. 1987; Bond, 1986; Burnard, 1989) and courses in these forms of training are frequently organized by women's groups, growth centres and extramural departments of colleges and universities.

In health care education and training, the use of video can enhance self-awareness by allowing students to view themselves from another person's point of view. Such training, however, should always be voluntary. Some people find the use of video taping a gross invasion of personal territory and the method should be used with discretion.

As we have noted, work on the body via Reichian bodywork, yoga, tai chi, the martial arts and sport all have their place in self-awareness development both for their effects on the body and for their limit-testing capacity. A quieter, more reflective approach is the use of journals or diaries and these can be used to monitor self-awareness development alongside educational development. Probably the ideal is a combination of a variety of approaches: introspection, with a group, active and passive. In this way, the self is studied in all its aspects and in a variety of contexts. As we have noted, the 'self' is not a static once-and-for-all thing but an entity that is constantly changing depending, among other things, on the people we are with. The combined approach is also healthier in that it encourages the combination of sport and exercise alongside meditation and more reflective practices. It also allows for normal social relationships to develop alongside periods of solidarity. No one ever became self-aware by shutting out the rest of the world. Also, it is important that self-awareness development has a practical end – the enhancement of interpersonal relationships and skills.

THE JOHARI WINDOW

Another approach to self-awareness development is via the use of the Johari Window (Luft, 1969). The window is illustrated in Fig. 3.2. There is nothing particularly mysterious about the name: it was named after the first names of its two authors, Harry Inghams and Joseph Luft! The window picks out four possible aspects of the self:

- The open area
- The blind area
- The hidden area
- The unknown area.

The open area is easily described. It is that part of us that *we* know about ourselves and that *others* know about us. Thus both I and my family know that I am fairly tall, reasonably hard working and rather moody. No particular secrets here!

The blind area is that part of us that *others* know about us but

	Known to self	Not known to self
Known to others	OPEN AREA	BLIND AREA
Not known to others	HIDDEN AREA	UNKNOWN AREA

Figure 3.2 The Johari Window.

of which we are unaware. Thus, my colleagues at work presumably have some opinions of me that I do not know and with which I can therefore neither agree nor disagree. I can only become aware of these 'blind' aspects as others disclose to me their view of me.

The hidden area contains all of those things that I do not tell others about. Thus, part of me remains hidden to others. It is notable that I am not hidden equally to all persons. There are people, such as my family, who know a lot about me and others, such as acquaintances, who know very little about me.

The unknown area is that hypothesized area that is unknown to me and to others. It remains uncharted territory. Luft's argument is simply this: we can learn more about our hidden selves if we disclose more of ourselves to others (Fig. 3.3) or receive feedback about ourselves from others (Fig. 3.4). Under the conditions of both self-disclosure and feedback from others, we can 'grow' considerably in the unknown area (Fig. 3.5). Luft argues that we can all enhance our sense of self and get to know ourselves and others better if we take the risk of disclosing ourselves and if we are prepared to hear other people's assessment of us.

In terms of stress, the model has much to commend it. If we are stressed and yet do not talk to others, we feel more stressed. We also remain 'hidden' to others. On the other hand, if we can talk about how we feel we can begin to feel some relief – sometimes *just because* we talk. Also, we can be reassured by listening to what others say of us. To hear other people's evaluation of us can give us a more realistic sense of self. And, anyway, it is

	Known to self	Not known to self
Known to others	OPEN AREA	BLIND AREA
Not known to others	HIDDEN AREA	UNKNOWN AREA

Figure 3.3 The Johari Window following self-disclosure

	Known to self	Not known to self
Known to others	OPEN AREA	BLIND AREA
Not known to others	HIDDEN AREA	UNKNOWN AREA

Figure 3.4 The Johari Window following feedback from others.

probably more comfortable to know what others think of us than to remain in the dark! In coming to know the 'hidden area' better, we also discover new strengths and resources.

SELF-AWARENESS AND THE HEALTH CARE PROFESSIONAL

Having explored the concept of self and examined some methods of self-awareness development, the question remains: 'Why develop self-awareness anyway?'

	Known to self	Not known to self
Known to others	OPEN AREA	BLIND AREA
Not known to others	HIDDEN AREA	UNKNOWN AREA

Figure 3.5 The Johari Window following both disclosure and feedback from others.

In the first instance, to discover more about ourselves is to differentiate ourselves from others. If we cannot differentiate between *our own* thoughts and feelings and those of others, we stand to blur our ego boundaries, our sense of ourself as an independent, autonomous being. Conversely, if we constantly blur the distinction between 'you and me' we risk not recognizing the other person's independence and autonomy. When ego boundaries are blurred, we loose the sense of whose problem is whose. With self-awareness we can learn to distinguish between our problems and those of others, and vice versa. This is particularly important in sensitive areas such as psychiatry and the care of the dying. Real involvement and care in these fields also involves (almost paradoxically) the ability to detach ourselves a little in order to see things in perspective. If we cannot engage in this distancing we risk being drawn into other people's problems to such a degree that we can no longer help them. *Their* problems have become *ours*.

To become self-aware is also to learn conscious use of the self. We become agents: we are able to choose to act rather than feel acted upon. We learn to select therapeutic interventions from a range of options so that the patient or client benefits more completely. If we are blind to ourselves we are also blind to our choices. We are blind, then, to caring and to therapeutic choices that we could make on behalf of our patients. The whole process of making interventions can become less stressful if we choose those interventions.

Once we can combine two aspects – differentiation from others and an increased awareness of the range of therapeutic choices available – we can be more sensitive to the needs and wants of others. We can even choose to *forget ourselves* in order to give ourselves more completely to others. No longer do we run the risk of getting sucked into other people's problems, nor do we confuse *our* thoughts and feelings with those of our patients. We can offer therapeutic distance with therapeutic choice. Stress in health care often comes about because the boundaries between us and our clients becomes blurred. Somehow, *their* problems become caught up with *our* problems. Self-awareness can help us to disentangle ourselves.

PROBLEMS IN SELF-AWARENESS DEVELOPMENT

It is worth repeating the point made at various stages throughout this chapter: the aim of self-awareness development is to enable us to increase our interpersonal skills and cope better with stress. The path to such awareness is, however, fraught with problems. First is the problem of egocentricity. It is possible to become caught up in the idea of understanding the self to the degree that it becomes an end in itself. This tends to lead to the person becoming self-indulgent and self-centred. Clearly such positions are not compatible with altruism or concern for others.

Second, it is possible for those who develop self-awareness to believe that they have discovered insights that set them apart from, or even make them better than, other people. A sign of such development is sometimes the loss of a sense of humour. Life becomes very earnest. True self-awareness, however, tends to lead to a lightness of touch and a sense of humility at the sheer vastness of the task in hand. To continue with that task, it is important that the person maintains (and exercises) a sense of humour in order to keep sight of the 'larger canvas'. Certainly the best run self-awareness groups are those that offer a 'light' atmosphere. If the atmosphere becomes too heavy and earnest, it is likely to put everyone off. It is certainly not conducive to easy and frank self-disclosure.

Linked to this is the problem of the self-awareness group facilitator becoming something of a 'guru' figure. As people find things out about themselves, they sometimes tend to imagine that the group facilitator has special qualities that allow this to happen. As a result, those people tend to view the facilitator up someone with unique abilities. Sometimes, too, the facilitator believes in this image and ends up acting out the role of guru. Again, caution and humility are keywords. Both group members and facilitator should remember that the facilitator is human, like everyone else.

Finally comes the issue of voluntariness. Self-awareness cannot be forced upon people. Facilitators of self-awareness groups would do well to exercise what Heron (1977) calls the voluntary principle. By this principle, invoked as the beginning of any self-awareness training course and repeated at intervals throughout such a course, no one at any time will have pressure exerted on them to take part and everyone who takes part in any exercise will do so of his or her own free will. If self-awareness is about developing autonomy and the exercise of choice, it is important that such autonomy and choice begins with people deciding whether or not a given exercise suits them at this time. Accepting and respecting other people's frailties, their reserve and their choice not to disclose aspects of themselves until they are ready, are all part of the process of facilitation. Such understanding on the part of the facilitator will do much to increase the confidence of group members and to create an atmosphere conducive to self-understanding.

SELF-AWARENESS AND STRESS REDUCTION

As we have noted above, developing self-awareness can enable us to develop a more caring, more sensitive and more appropriate approach to patient care. It can also help us to monitor our stress levels. In the next chapter we explore some specific exercises for developing self-awareness and thus for helping to cope with and overcome stress.

SUMMARY

Self-awareness is essential to the process of coping with stress. This chapter has explored the notion of self-awareness from various theoretical perspectives. It has also examined ways in which the health professional can develop self-awareness both as the means of enhancing therapeutic competence and as a practical method of coping with stress. We must first know that we are stressed before we can deal with it.

4

Self-awareness activities for stress reduction

Sometimes I need to be totally by myself, away from anyone who can make claims on my time: even for just a few minutes.
Student physiotherapist

Aims of this Chapter

This chapter explores:

• Ways of reducing stress through self-awareness
• Gestalt-based activities for stress reduction.

SELF-AWARENESS AND STRESS REDUCTION

Self-awareness has been discussed as a means of helping to cope with and overcome stress. Self-awareness can help us to realize the following:

• We can appreciate our 'ego boundaries' – the points at which 'I' end and 'you' begin. Thus, it can help us to be clear about problems that belong to our clients and problems that are our own. It can help us to maintain an optimal psychological distance in relation to our clients: neither so close that we are over-involved, nor so far that we are unable to appreciate fully our clients' problems.
• We can monitor ourselves. As we begin to notice our actions and reactions, we are better able to *choose* certain lines of actions. Rather than feeling acted upon, we are able to be the

initiators of action: we begin to take responsibility for what we do.

- We can notice when we are reaching our limits. Rather than pushing on regardless, we can begin to choose to slow down, to rest, to change direction or to engage in other behaviour. Without self-awareness, we can be 'blind' to our own actions.
- We can notice physical and psychological changes. If we are not particularly self-aware, we lose touch with ourselves, both physically and psychologically. We no longer notice what is happening to our bodies. We no longer notice whether or not we are particularly fit or unfit. Nor do we tend to notice our changing moods. Self-awareness can enable us to take care of our physical fitness and can help to prevent burnout in that we take more notice of our psychological status.

This chapter offers a series of exercises that can be used to enhance self-awareness based on techniques used in gestalt therapy.

Stress in Health Care: a Case in Point 5

Andrew Duncan works as a lecturer in health studies at a large polytechnic. He is eager to progress in the academic field and begins to take on various accept a variety of consultancies for local organizations. Those consultancies involve helping to set up 'Look After Yourself' courses for employees of small companies. He also begins to write papers and articles for journals.

As he develops his career, so his marriage begins to show signs of strain. His wife complains that he is often away from home and that he tends to bring more and more work home with him. As a result of this tension at home, he throws himself more and more into work and finds himself becoming less and less effective. He is a victim of the 'busy syndrome'.

A colleague and friend suggests to Duncan that he seeks help through the local RELATE (marriage guidance) organization. After some weeks, Duncan and his wife are able to talk through their respective positions with a RELATE counsellor and are able to reassess their lives. Duncan realizes that his addiction to work has made him and his marriage highly stressed and he is able to make

the necessary adjustments. In the future, he agrees to limit
the amount of 'outside' work that he takes on and agrees
not to bury himself in work at home. Duncan's marriage
survives.

GESTALT THERAPY

'Gestalt' is a German word for which there is no absolute English
translation. It roughly means 'form'. Gestalt therapy, an important influence in the humanistic approach to experiential learning,
is a true mind/body therapy, aiming to integrate both aspects of
the person. This is done by helping the individual to become
aware of both psychological and physiological events as they
happen. Thus it has a 'here and now' focus. Gestalt therapy is
only interested in the individual's past in as much as it affects
present-moment awareness. In an important sense, the present is
all there is. The past is past and cannot be brought back, the
future is yet to come and can only be speculated upon. The person
who can live more fully in the present is more likely to notice,
live and learn more fully.

Fritz Perls (1969a,b), a psychoanalyst, developed this therapeutic approach, drawing from psychoanalysis itself, Reichian
character analysis theory, existential philosophy and Eastern
philosophy. By all accounts he was a charismatic person who no
doubt developed his theory in his own, idiosyncratic style. Gestalt
draws from psychoanalytical theory many beliefs about 'unconscious' or unrecognized factors at work in our minds and bodies.
One of its aims, like many other therapies, is to make the unconscious conscious. It develops Reich's (1949) work on the concept
of trapped emotion in the body's musculature (or what Reich
called 'character armour'). Reich believed that we carry our
repressed emotions around with us in our muscle clusters. Thus
people who consistently refuse to face their own anger often carry
the anger around with them in the neck and shoulder muscles.
You may want to check the status of *your own* muscle clusters
and notice to what degree you continuously tense certain muscle
groups.

Gestalt is an existential approach in that it encourages the
individual to take full responsibility for his or her actions, and
acknowledge that it is *we* as individuals who invest our lives with
meaning. Finally, it borrows from Eastern philosophy a fasci-

nation with paradox. Thus it is paradoxical that we often say exactly the opposite of what we really mean. e.g. 'I'm perfectly relaxed' or 'It was so nice to see you again'. Again, apply this principle to yourself. How often do you say exactly the opposite of what you mean?

Perls' gestalt therapy combined all these influences to create a type of therapy that *encouraged* feelings rather than resisted them. In many other therapies, for example, the client would he helped to *oppose* any feelings. Thus the anxious person was encouraged to relax. Perls' method was to encourage the person to *experience* anxiety and, if necessary, increase it. Paradoxically, as this happened, the person very often relaxed and felt more comfortable. Release was acquired through acceptance and experience of the emotion. After all, the anxious person is very good at feeling anxious, and gestalt therapy, instead of fighting that inclination, allows it. Perls maintained that it is not until we fully accept ourselves *as we are* (and not as we would wish to be or think we ought to be) that change can come about. Further, he noted that we often blame others for our predicament ('if it wasn't for my mother . . . I would be quite different') or we appeal to some dubious theory about the nature of our make up ('I can't help it . . . it's the way I'm made!'). Gestalt therapy aims at helping the individual to experience and to *own* those experiences.

As with many humanistic therapies, gestalt therapy tends to use the following 'ground rules' during practise. Gestalt therapist often prefer their clients to:

(a) use 'I' rather than 'you', 'we' or 'people' – thus, 'I am unhappy at the moment' rather than 'you know what it's like, you tend to get unhappy at times like this';
(b) talk to others directly, in the 'first person', rather than indirectly – thus, 'I don't agree with what you are saying' rather than 'I didn't agree with what Kevin said';
(c) avoid asking questions, particularly 'why' questions; it is better to listen for the statement behind the question – thus, 'I am hurt by what you say' rather than 'Why are you saying that?'.
(d) remain, as far as possible, in the present rather than slipping into reminiscences.

These ground rules are valuable in helping the individual and the group to remain fully in the present and to take responsibility for their own thoughts, feelings and actions. They are also a useful set of guidelines for clear communication in *any* setting. It may well be that stress is reduced through the use of such ground rules in everyday communication. If we can be more clear about what it is we want to say and how we are to say it, we are likely to decrease our anxiety and tension – at least in the long term. Initially, the use of the ground rules may *increase* tension, for many of us are not used to communicating so directly.

The gestalt therapist works by helping the client to become more aware of verbal expressions, tones of voice, body movements, gestures and so forth. Such a therapist does not interpret or offer explanations of what the client is saying but encourages the client to verbalize his or her own insights. The aim of therapy is to increase self-awareness and self-understanding through moment-to-moment observation. It encourages people to take full responsibility for themselves and to realize that, as 'authors' of their own lives, they are free to exercise choice. In this respect, the gestalt process is similar to the co-counselling process. Both are non-interpretative and both emphasize the freedom of the individual.

The gestalt approach offers the health professional an alternative way of supporting patients and colleagues. If the health professional can *allow* the patient or colleague to experience such feelings as anxiety, unhappiness, loneliness as well as the more positive feelings, then (according to gestalt theory) those feelings may change. Many health professionals have become compulsive carers and many believe that their aim should always be the reduction of negative feelings in the people they meet. Perhaps to allow such feelings is not only to allow the individuals to grow but also to allow them to develop ways of coping with such feelings in the future.

The exercises that follow are based on approaches and activities used in gestalt therapy. Take your time over them. Do them slowly and deliberately rather than rush through them at one sitting. If taken slowly, they can enhance your self-awareness and thus lower your stress levels by helping you to get to know yourself better and to accept yourself as you are – warts and all! Be wary of just reading them through. You need to try them as you read.

SELF-AWARENESS EXERCISES

EXERCISE 1

Aim of the exercise: to explore your visual field

Activity: Sit quietly and look around you. Allow your focus of attention to come to rest on various things in the room. Pay attention to each item and explore every aspect of it. As you move on to the next object, notice the differences between this object and the previous one in terms of colour, texture, shape and so forth.

EXERCISE 2

Aim of the exercise: to explore your senses

Activity: Allow your attention to focus on your hearing. Just sit and notice the sounds you can hear and the variety of them. Try to identify and name each of them. As you do this, notice what happens to your *other* senses. Notice, too, how long you can sustain this concentration on one particular sense. You can also try this exercise with other senses.

EXERCISE 3

Aim of the exercise: to explore your focus of attention

Activity: Sit quietly for a few minutes, breathing deeply. Now allow yourself to notice the focus of your attention. It may, for instance, start by being focused on your breathing. It may then shift to an aspect of the room in which you are sitting. Just allow your focus of attention to shift gently but *notice* it as it shifts. Do not attempt to control your attention: simply be aware of where your attention goes. Again, notice how long you can sustain this concentration on your focus of attention.

EXERCISE 4

Aim of the exercise: to explore things that you choose NOT *to focus on.*

Activity: Bearing in mind the last exercise, notice the sorts of things that you did *not* focus on. Did you, for instance, avoid focusing on certain thoughts? Did you avoid looking at certain things? Did you avoid certain noises that you thought might be distracting? As you explore these objects or sensations that you previously avoided, allow yourself to focus on them completely and notice how you feel as you do this. What do you *frequently* avoid focusing on in your life?

EXERCISE 5

Aim of the exercise: to explore your breathing

Activity: Sit quietly and focus your attention on your breathing. Do not attempt to change it in any way. Just notice it. How do you breathe? Are your breaths deep, shallow, rapid, slow? Do you sigh a lot? Does your breathing rate change as you focus on it? Again, consider how your breathing changes in everyday life. What is your everyday breathing like?

Now allow yourself to breathe more deeply. What happens to the rest of your body as you do this? Pay attention to your stomach, your chest and the muscles around your shoulders as your breathing alters and notice any changes in these areas.

EXERCISE 6

Aim of the exercise: to explore your thinking

Activity: Sit quietly and allow your attention to focus on your thoughts. Observe yourself thinking. Do not attempt to think about anything in particular; instead, merely notice the ebb and flow of your thoughts. Do your thoughts circle around one particular issue? Does your thinking hop from one topic to another? Just notice when one thought starts and how your mind deals with that thought. As you do this exercise, notice any changes in your breathing and in the rest of your body as your thoughts change.

EXERCISE 7

Aim of the exercise: to explore topics that you avoid thinking about

Activity: This exercise is more difficult. Sit quietly and focus your attention on your thoughts. This time, allow yourself to notice any sorts of thoughts that you would normally *avoid*. Then allow those thoughts to take shape. Notice what happens to your breathing and to the rest of your body as you do this. Notice any tensions that occur as a result of your thoughts.

Now shift your attention, fairly rapidly, from those thoughts that you normally avoid to thoughts that are more pleasant or more acceptable. Notice the changes that take place in your breathing and in your body as this occurs.

EXERCISE 8

Aim of the exercise: to explore shuttling your attention between your thoughts and the outside world

Activity: Sit quietly and allow your attention to focus on your thoughts. Do not try to control them in any way but allow yourself to notice how those thoughts ebb and flow. Once you have been doing this for a few minutes, open your eyes and focus your attention on one particular object in the room. Consciously redirect your focus of attention from your thoughts to the object. As you make this switch, notice any changes in your breathing and in the rest of your body. Notice any tendency for your body to become more or less tense. Now allow your attention to remain focused on the object and explore every aspect of it. Once you have done this for a few minutes, close your eyes and allow your attention to switch back to your thoughts. Notice any changes in your body and notice, too, if you experience any difficulty in switching attention in this way. Notice whether or not you find focusing 'inwards' or 'outwards' more difficult.

EXERCISE 9

Aim of the exercise: to explore your approach to these exercises

Activity: Sit quietly and notice how you *feel* about doing these exercises, so far. Are you trying hard to do them properly? Are you doing them in a slightly cynical frame of mind? Are they making you angry? Do you find them relaxing? Do not dismiss any of these feelings but allow them to emerge fully. Now ask yourself: 'On what occasions have I felt these sorts of feelings before?' Spend a little time exploring the feelings and thoughts that emerge as a result of this activity.

EXERCISE 10

Aim of the exercise: to explore awareness of the body

Activity: Allow yourself to notice any sensations in your body. Let your attention move from one part of your body to another and notice how each part feels. Are there some parts that are tense while others are relaxed? Does your breathing change as your attention moves its focus? Now allow yourself to *exaggerate* any sensation that you notice. If there is tension, increase it; if you are moving your arm or leg slightly, increase that movement. Now notice how you can take responsibility for how your body feels and that you can *choose* to relax or tense many aspects of your body. Notice those parts of the body that are fairly constantly tense.

Now reverse the procedure. Pay attention to those parts of the body in which you exaggerated a sensation and try to reverse the procedure. Thus, try to relax those parts that are tense. Stop any movement in your arms and legs. Notice what happens as you allow yourself to stop.

EXERCISE 11

Aim of the exercise: to explore your physical movements in everyday life

Activity: Choose a fairly mundane activity such as cleaning your teeth or opening an envelope. First, carry out the activity at normal speed and *notice* how you do it. Notice the amount of energy that you put into the activity and notice what muscle clusters are involved. Then, slow the activity to about half speed and notice what happens. Then try the activity again, using less effort to carry out the task. Allow yourself to notice yourself 'in action' on frequent occasions throughout the day and practice reducing the effort taken to complete various tasks. Notice when everyday tasks seem to take more effort and when they are easy to carry out. Make a note of how you are feeling when these changes occur.

EXERCISE 12

Aim of the exercise: to explore your surroundings

Activity: This is a useful activity for distracting yourself when you are under pressure or feeling particularly tense.

At some point during the day, when you are walking from one place to another or when you are just 'out for a walk', focus your attention, completely, on what is going on around you. Allow yourself to notice everything that comes into view. Notice, also, the colours, sounds, movements and so forth. Do not attempt to focus on one particular event or object but allow your attention to range over everything that is in your visual path. Notice, as you do this, how much you *usually* do *not* notice about your surroundings. Notice, too, how this activity can allow you to distance yourself from the thoughts that usually pre-occupy you. This 'walking meditation' or exercise to focus the attention outside of yourself can be used consciously whenever you need some breathing space between you and what is worrying you.

EXERCISE 13

Aim of the exercise: to explore your self-image

Activity: Sit quietly and close your eyes. Now imagine that you are looking at yourself, sitting in front of you. Form an image of yourself as you imagine yourself to be. Notice what you see. Do you like the image? Is the image as you expected it would be? Do you compare yourself to others? Is the comparison favourable or unfavourable?

EXERCISE 14

Aim of the exercise: to explore your relationship with yourself

Activity: Sit and imagine that you are looking at yourself, sitting in front of you. Now tell yourself (silently) what you should and should not do. Start each sentence with 'You should . . .' or 'You should not . . .'. Listen to yourself as you do this. Are you judgemental. . . . accepting. . . . highly critical? What does this exercise tell you about your relationship with yourself?

EXERCISE 15

Aim of the exercise: to explore coping with self-criticism

Activity: Repeat the first part of the previous exercise. Sit and imagine that you are sitting in front of yourself. Now tell yourself what you should not do. Start each sentence with 'You should not . . .'. Now respond to each of those statements. Again, notice the *tone* of your response. Notice any tendency to justify your position, to disregard the 'critical' part of you or to ignore it. Practice switching between the critical part of yourself and the part that answers that criticism. Notice which part feels more comfortable or which part gets the upper hand. What does this tell you about your self-criticism and your defensiveness? Are you as critical with others as you are with yourself . . . more so . . .

less so? Should the criticisms you level at others also be levelled at yourself?

EXERCISE 16

Aim of the exercise: to explore the present

Activity: If you have been doing two or three of these exercises, stop, close your eyes and just notice what is happening to you. Notice the thoughts that are going through your mind. Notice your feelings. Notice the status of your body in terms of relaxation or tension. Now compare those thoughts, feelings and bodily sensations with those you had prior to starting the exercises. Return to this exercise frequently while working through these activities. Try to return to it during the course of a working day and explore your current cognitive, affective and physical status. Notice how you can *modify* that status if you can become aware of it. Too often we are so taken up with what we are doing that we are unable to notice how we are thinking or feeling.

EXERCISE 17

Aim of the exercise: to explore the way you talk to other people

Activity: Sit quietly and close your eyes. Now bring to mind a person with whom you have frequent contact. Have an imaginary conversation with that person. Continue this conversation for about a minute. Now listen to yourself. Notice your tone of voice, the content of your speech, whether or not you are open and relaxed or quiet and defensive.

Now imagine that another person has joined you. Switch the conversation to that person. Notice the change in your tone, content and status with regard to that person. Continue *that* conversation for about a minute before switching back to the first person. Notice how you feel at the *moment* of switching back. Check your thinking, your feelings and your physical status.

Now let yourself imagine a third conversation, this time with the person you feel *most comfortable with*. Notice how your tone, manner, thoughts, feelings and physical status change again. Explore what it is about this person that makes it so easy to talk to him or her. Now notice any similarities between this person and yourself. Finish the activity by exploring any thoughts or associations that you have during the exercise.

EXERCISE 18

Aim of the exercise: exploring the past

Activity: Sit quietly with your eyes closed. Let your mind drift back to the past. First of all, go back about five years. What is it that comes to mind? Is the memory pleasant or unpleasant? Do you enjoy the process of recalling the past? What are the worst and best things about the process?

Now go back about ten years and consider the pros and cons of that memory, noting, as you go, whether or not the memory is pleasant or unpleasant. Repeat the activity, going back a further five years each time until you are as far back as you can remember.

Finally, switch between that earliest memory and the present time . . . then back again. Notice, as you do this switching, the thoughts and feelings that accompany the switch. Is it an easy process to carry out? What happens to your body as you do this? Reflect on the degree to which you live in the present and the degree to which you live in the past. Notice whether or not you tend to think that the past was 'better' than the present. Notice the difference, in terms of stress, between 'then' and 'now'. Were you less or more stressed in the past? Are the things that caused you stress then still the things that cause you stress today?

EXERCISE 19

Aim of the exercise: to explore your relationship with your parents

Activity: Sit quietly with your eyes closed. Now imagine one of your parents sitting in front of you. Notice *which* parent you choose. Notice how the parent looks as he or she sits in front of you. Notice how you feel as the parent sits there.

Now reflect on what you want to say to that parent, given that you can say anything you like. Do you want to be critical . . . encouraging . . . positive . . . negative? Now consider what it is (or what it was) that stops you saying those things to that parent.

Now imagine your other parent sitting in front of you. What is the difference in your feelings now that *this* parent is in front of you? What do you want to say to him or her? Which parent is easier to talk to?

EXERCISE 20

Aim of the exercise: to explore fears and needs

Activity: Sit with your eyes closed. Now make a series of statements that begin 'I'm afraid to . . .' (followed by immediate completion of the statement). Then make a series of statements that begin 'I'd like to . . .'. Which is the longer list? What differences are there between the two, or are the lists related? Does one particular topic recur? Explore the implications of these two lists and identify what you must do to overcome the fears and satisfy the needs.

EXERCISE 21

Aim of the exercise: to explore likes and dislikes

Activity: Allow your attention to focus on the environment around you. Let it focus on particular objects. As you contemplate each object, say to yourself, 'I like . . . about this object' followed by, 'I dislike . . . about this object'. Once you have done this, move on to another object and repeat the process. Notice the similarities and differences between what you like and dislike about the things around you. Notice, too, when you react very strongly for or against something. Experiment with *changing* the way you label things. For an object that you dislike, try pretending, temporarily, that you like it. Then make the statements, 'I like . . . about this object' and 'I dislike . . . about this object'. What changes in your perception occurs as a result of this change? What does all this tell you about how you judge things? Do you make similar sorts of judgements about *people*?

Practical Methods of Coping with Stress in the Health Professions: 4

THOUGHT STOPPING

Sometimes, stress can lead to circular thinking. Our thoughts go round and round a particular (usually unpleasant) topic without anything getting resolved in the process. One way of dealing with this is to consciously choose to think of other things. One aid to this can be to take a deep breath and to say STOP! The 'stop', in this case, becomes the necessary injunction to move on mentally to another topic.

SUMMARY

This chapter has offered a series of exercises in developing self-awareness as an approach to stress reduction. The activities described here can be followed through with others available from a variety of sources (Perls *et al.*, 1951; Canfield and Wells, 1976; Ernst and Goodison, 1981; Roet, 1989).

5

Stress and relaxation

You have to go a long way to beat a good book, a gin and
tonic and a long hot bath!

Nurse teacher

Aims of this chapter

This chapter explores:

• The nature of stress and relaxation
• Breathing techniques
• Relaxation activities.

THE NATURE OF STRESS AND RELAXATION

Stress often manifests itself most clearly in the form of physical
tension. Whatever the cause of the stress, if we can learn to relax
it follows that we are likely to feel relief from stress, at least in
the short term. That is not to oversimplify the situation nor to
suggest that relaxation, alone, can cure stress. It is merely to note
that by learning to physically relax we can better prepare ourselves
for dealing with the practical problems that are often associated
with stress. The opposite is also true: if we are physically tense,
we are less likely to be able to solve problems effectively, for that
tension also has its effects on our psychological state. Physical
tension leads to loss of concentration, anxiety and self-doubt.

It is suggested that relaxation methods are always combined
with practical problem-solving methods that attempt to address

the stressor. Trying to remove the source of stress seems a better idea than only attempting to stay calm in an impossible situation. On the other hand, there are many occasions on which we have to learn to live with stress. Certainly, in the health professions, most of us face stressful situations daily that *cannot* easily be 'solved'. Again, in this situation, it seems likely that if we can learn to relax physically we are more likely to be able to live with the things that cannot be changed.

Stress in Health Care: a Case in Point 6

Angela Smith is an occupational therapist who works in a rehabilitation unit which cares for people with long-term psychiatric and emotional problems. She finds herself drawn to depressive patients who find, in turn, that they can talk to her.

*As a result of continual close involvement with people who question the validity of life and who are at the end of their tether, Angela finds that **she** is questioning **her own** reasons for living. She experiences a period of dispiritedness and inability to invest life with meaning. She finds that she goes to work and operates on 'automatic pilot', with little real enthusiasm for what she does.*

*Eventually, she is invited by a friend to a local church group. She visits this but finds that she is unable to accept the teaching that is offered there. The group **does** however encourage her to clarify her own beliefs and values. Slowly, Angela works out her own belief system and this, in turn, enables her to work with renewed interest. She realizes, too, that her particular interest in helping depressed people was linked with her **own** need to find meaning. As she clarifies her own beliefs and values, she begins to experience less stress.*

The activities that are described here are simple methods of learning to relax. They range from simple breathing exercises, through relaxation 'scripts' to exercises in imagery. They can be used by health professionals working alone or in small groups. While some prefer to use them, independently, at home, others will find benefit from carrying out these exercises in a small group. If you are planning to set up a stress-reduction group, the following points should be borne in mind:

- Choose a room that is quiet, warm and free from interruptions.
- If you are working with a 'script', read it through slowly but in a 'normal' voice. Do not try to be particularly 'soothing' and never try to be 'hypnotic' in your tone: such affectations rarely work!
- Allow people time to rouse themselves afterwards. Do not rush to finish a relaxation group. Allow plenty of time for rousing and coming round after the activity. Plan this time into the structure of the group.
- Allow people to discuss the experience afterwards. This can help people to learn from each other. It can also give you useful tips about how to modify or adapt future sessions in line with people's needs and wants.
- Consider rotating the leadership of a stress-reduction group. In this way, no one becomes too dependent on anyone else and everyone gets an equal chance to learn to relax physically.

What can relaxation activities do? According to Kitzinger (1979) and McCaffery (1979), relaxation activities may be used to:

- decrease anxiety;
- assist in stress management;
- promote sleep;
- reduce pain or the perception of pain;
- alleviate muscle tension;
- warm or cool parts of the body;
- decrease blood pressure;
- slow the heartbeat;
- combat fatigue;
- reduce or prevent the physiological and psychological effects of stress;
- serve as a coping device or skill;
- enhance the effectiveness of pain relief measures.

BREATHING TECHNIQUES

The 'breathing square' (Wallace, 1989) offers a useful and simple method of controlling tension and reducing stress. You are asked to visualize a square as illustrated in Fig. 5.1. Each side of the square has a time value allocated to it. All you do is work around the four sides of the square, paying attention to the instructions

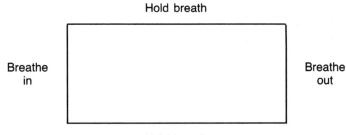

Figure 5.1 The breathing square.

and adhering to the time values. The activity calms down any tendency towards over-breathing, regulates the pace of breathing and distracts the mind from other thoughts. In this last respect, it is similar to some of the meditational practices described in the next chapter. A variant of this practice is to work around the four sides of the television screen, according to the schedule of instructions and time, as an aid to further relaxation while sitting down at home.

Another breathing exercise that is simple to teach or learn is described by Davis *et al.* (1982) as follows:

Lie down on the floor with knees bent and spine straight. Scan body for tension. Inhale slowly and deeply, feeling your abdomen slightly rise with each inhalation. Inhale through your nose and exhale gently through your mouth making a relaxing whooshing sound. Continue deep breathing for 5–10 minutes, focus on the sound of your breath, the gentle rise and fall of your abdomen and the deepening sense of relaxation. Let other thoughts or distractions pass in and out of your mind. Practise daily and use whenever you feel tension.

Practical Methods of Coping with Stress in the Health Professions: 5

ASSERT YOURSELF

It is easy, when stressed, to be subservient to the needs of others. Woodcock and Francis (1982) suggest that research indicates that assertive people tend to:

- *Avoid confused emotions.*

- *Be simple in their dealings with others.*
- *Carry through what they set out to do.*
- *Not put themselves down.*
- *Watch out for 'flack'.*
- *Acknowledge that error does not weaken.*
- *Go out to win.*

RELAXATION ACTIVITIES

Relaxation script 1

This script encourages you to relax by focusing on separate sets of muscles and by progressively relaxing those muscles.

Lie on your back, with you hands by your sides . . . stretch your legs out and have your feet about a foot apart . . . pay attention to your breathing . . . take two or three really deep breaths . . . breathing in through your nose and out through your mouth . . . now allow your head to sink into the floor . . . your head is sinking into the floor and you begin to feel more and more relaxed . . . allow your brow to become smooth and relaxed . . . feel your cheeks relaxing . . . let your jaw drop and relax . . . feel the tension draining out of your temples as your jaw relaxes . . . let yourself relax . . . more and more . . . let your shoulders drop and feel your neck and shoulders relax . . . more and more relaxed . . . now become aware of your right arm . . . let your right arm become heavy and warm and relaxed . . . your upper right arm . . . lower arm . . . your right hand . . . the whole of your right arm is heavy and warm and relaxed . . . no tension . . . just relaxed . . . now become aware of your left arm . . . let your left arm become heavy and warm and relaxed . . . your upper left arm . . . lower arm . . . your left hand feels heavy and warm and relaxed . . . the whole of your left arm is heavy and warm and relaxed . . . your shoulders and chest feel relaxed . . . your abdomen feels relaxed . . . your pelvis and hips . . . you're feeling heavy and warm and relaxed . . . your right leg and foot feels heavy and relaxed . . . your left leg feels the same . . . your whole body is relaxed . . . no tension . . . just relaxed . . . and you can appreciate what if feels like to feel safe and warm and relaxed . . . just lie back and enjoy the feeling.

Now, slowly, stretch yourself . . . stretch your arms and

legs . . . your toes and fingers . . . now slowly sit up . . . taking your time . . . slowly sit up and take a few deep breaths . . . and appreciate what it feels like to feel really relaxed.

Relaxation script 2

This script encourages you to imagine what it feels like *inside* your body and to relax almost from the 'inside out'!

Lie on your back with your hands by your sides . . . stretch your legs out and have your feet about a foot apart . . . pay attention to your breathing . . . take two or three deep breaths . . . breathe in through the nose . . . and out through the mouth . . . now let your breathing become gentle and relaxed . . . now I want you to become aware of your body . . . starting at the toes . . . try to experience the feeling in your feet and toes . . . try to experience that as though you were *inside* your feet and toes . . . now become aware of the lower parts of your legs . . . as if from the inside . . . now your knees . . . become aware of your joints . . . become aware of your thighs and the top of your legs . . . experience them as if you were inside them . . . now experience you pelvis and hips . . . now your abdomen . . . as if from the inside . . . put your attention into your chest . . . experience the feeling inside your chest . . . now your hands . . . your lower arms . . . your upper arms . . . imagine being inside your arms . . . now experience your shoulders . . . feel the shoulder joints . . . experience the feeling inside your neck . . . the back of your head . . . now your head itself . . . feel and experience your face . . . the muscles in your face . . . your lips . . . your nose . . . your eyes . . . finally . . . your scalp . . . imagine the feelings as though you were beneath your scalp . . . remaining fully aware of all parts of your body . . . notice which parts you can fully experience . . . and which parts are numb to you . . . see if you can become more aware of those parts of your body . . . now just lie and relax for a few more moments . . . take a couple of deep breaths . . . and slowly . . . in your own time . . . sit up and open your eyes.

Relaxation script 3

This script asks you to make statements to yourself that encourage you to relax progressively. These instructions can be used at any time to relax a particular set of muscles or to encourage total relaxation.

Lie on your back or sit in a comfortable chair. Take one or two deep breaths, breathing in through the nose and out through the mouth. Now focus your attention on your head and say to yourself . . . 'my forehead is smooth and relaxed' . . . now focus on your scalp and say to yourself . . . 'my scalp and the back of my neck are becoming more and more relaxed'. Now move your attention to your shoulders and say to yourself . . . 'my shoulders have dropped and feel heavy and relaxed'. Now focus on your right arm and say to yourself . . . 'my right arm is heavy and relaxed . . . my right hand is warm and heavy and relaxed'. Now focus on your left arm and say to yourself . . . 'my left arm is heavy and relaxed . . . my left hand is warm and heavy and relaxed'. Now allow your attention to move to your stomach and abdomen and say to yourself . . . 'my stomach is relaxed . . . all the muscles are smooth and relaxed'. Finally, move your attention to each of your legs and say to yourself . . . 'my right leg is heavy and relaxed . . . my right foot feels heavy and warm and relaxed' . . . 'my left leg is heavy and relaxed . . . my left foot feels heavy and warm and relaxed'. Allow yourself to lay or sit quietly, breathing deeply and noticing what it feels like to feel completely relaxed.

Relaxation script 4

This is a short script that can be used at any time once you have learned the basic principles of relaxing sets of muscles.

Lie on the floor, flat on your back or sit in a comfortable chair. Take one or two deep breaths, breathing in through the nose and out through the mouth. Then focus your attention on different parts of your body, in turn. As your attention moves to each part, allow it to relax. Thus, say to yourself . . . 'head . . . shoulders . . . right arm . . . left arm . . . stomach and abdomen . . . right leg . . . left leg . . . right foot . . . left foot . . .

whole body'. As your attention shifts to each part of the body, allow that part to relax completely.

Relaxation script 5

This script takes a different approach. It encourages you first to *tense* your muscles before you relax them. This allows you to feel the difference between tense and relaxed muscles.

Lie on the floor, flat on your back, with your feet about a foot apart and with your hands resting by your side. Begin by gently breathing in through your nose and out through your mouth. Now put your attention into the muscles of your face and screw up all the muscles in your face as tight as you can. Hold that tension for just a few moments . . . then relax. Now focus on the muscles in your shoulders. Hunch your shoulders up as high as you can . . . hold the tension in them for a few moments . . . and relax, allowing your shoulders to drop and allowing your shoulders to broaden and make greater contact with the floor. Now clench both fists . . . tightly . . . then stretch both your arms downwards, towards your feet . . . hold the tension for just a few moments . . . and allow your hands and arms to relax completely. Then focus your attention on the muscles in your stomach. Take a deep breath and as you breathe out . . . allow the muscles of your stomach to be pulled in. Hold the tension for just a few moments . . . then relax them completely and breathe normally. . . . allow yourself to feel more and more relaxed. Finally, focus your attention on your legs and feet. Point both feet downwards as far as you can . . . allow your legs to push forward as far as you can . . . hold the tension for a few moments . . . then relax both legs and feet. Allow yourself to relax completely. Feel how much heavier your body now is and and allow your body to sink further into the floor. Appreciate what it feels like to have all your muscles relaxed. Breathe gently and easily and remain in the relaxed position for a few minutes.

Bernstein and Borkovec (1973) suggest concentrating on particular sets of muscles groups, in order. Their list of the groups to concentrate on are:

1. Dominant hand and forearm: make a tight fist.

2. Dominant biceps: push elbows down against the arm of the chair.
3. Non-dominant hand and forearm.
4. Non-dominant biceps.
5. Forehead: lift eyebrows.
6. Upper cheeks and nose: squint eyes and wrinkle nose.
7. Lower cheeks and jaws: bite down and pull corners of the mouth back.
8. Neck and throat: pull chin downwards without touching the chest.
9. Chest, shoulders and upper back: deep breath, hold and pull shoulder blades back.
10. Abdominal region: make stomach hard.
11. Dominant thigh: push back knee into chair.
12. Dominant calf: flex foot inward, point towards head.
13. Dominant foot: turn foot inward, point and curl toes.
14. Non-dominant thigh.
15. Non-dominant calf.
16. Non-dominant foot.

While working through this list, it is important to notice the tension in the various muscle clusters and then to release that tension. The list is best talked through by a colleague until you have memorized the sequence.

Finally, in this section, the technique developed by Benson from his work on the 'relaxation response' and developed by Benson's group at Harvard University's Thordike Memorial Laboratory (Benson, 1975). Benson's set of instructions for relaxation are:

1. Sit quietly in a comfortable position.
2. Close your eyes.
3. Deeply relax all your muscles, beginning at your feet and progressing up to your face. Keep them relaxed.
4. Breathe through your nose. Become aware of your breathing. As you breath out, say the word 'one', silently to yourself . . . Breathe easily and naturally.
5. Continue for 10 to 20 minutes. You may open your eyes to check the time, but do not use an alarm. When you finish, sit quietly for several minutes, at first with your eyes closed and later with your eyes open. Do not stand up for a few minutes.

6. Do not worry about whether you are successful in achieving a deep level of relaxation. Maintain a passive attitude and permit relaxation to occur at its own pace. When distracting thoughts occur, try to ignore them by not dwelling on them and return to repeating 'one'. Practise the technique once or twice daily, but not within two hours after any meal.

Benson's approach is typically the 'no-nonsense' approach to relaxation. He neither tries to mystify the process nor insists that you *must* relax. Indeed, how *could* you be implored to relax? The idea is a contradiction in terms.

SUMMARY

Breathing and relaxation activities make up one approach to coping with stress. This chapter has offered a variety of ways of controlling or modifying breathing and a number of approaches to relaxation. Those methods can be used by the health professional working alone or in a group. The activities described in this chapter can also be used with individual clients or as part of a relaxation programme in a group.

6

Stress, values and meditation

Examining sources of stress in detail with others often makes me feel worse. I prefer to do this alone. Then I can talk to myself, cry, be angry, uninhibited and then work through my feelings. I don't expect people to know exactly how I'm feeling.

Nurse

Aims of this chapter

This chapter explores:

● The need for meaning
● Spirituality and the search for meaning
● Personal values
● Meditation.

THE NEED FOR MEANING

The need to find meaning in what we do is very strong. It is probably the case that all human beings have to find meaning or face the problem of becoming dispirited. The question is often raised: '*Why* do certain things happen to us in the way they do?' This quest for meaning often becomes more acute in times of specific (and sometimes life-threatening) difficulty. The health professional often has to help people who are working through life-crises. The mere fact of being with people in this way can raise questions of meaning for the carer. The fact of being involved in other people's crises can also raise questions of meaning. The health professional who has to face the death of a client may well be tempted to raise the same sorts of 'why?' questions as did the client.

Helping other people to find meaning and searching for meaning ourselves can both be stressful activities. Finding a framework for making sense of life can also be problematic. Such frameworks often manifest themselves in very different sorts of ways. For some, a set of religious precepts helps in the process of making sense of life. For others, a philosophical, political or psychological set of beliefs and values is what helps to add meaning.

Perhaps the most stressful situation of all is the fact of having an inability to find meaning at all. Such a state may be described as *dispiritedness*. Dispiritedness, then, is the fact of being unable to invest life with meaning. It is sometimes, but not always, combined with depression. When it is not, it is characterized by a general sense of loss, a lack of conviction in what one is doing and a lack of enthusiasm for life in general. It may also be accompanied by a sense of cynicism and by the development of 'gallows humour'.

Some commentators have gone further and formally defined the notion of spiritual distress. Kim *et al.* (1987) define spiritual distress as

. . . distress of the human spirit . . . a disruption in the life principle which pervades a person's entire being and which integrates and transcends one's biological and psychosocial nature.

It may be argued, in passing, that the first part of this definition is tautological and that the second raises questions about what we are to understand by the idea of 'the life principle'. Kim *et al.* (1987) go on to offer defining characteristics of spiritual distress. According to them, spiritual distress:

- expresses concern with the meaning of life/death or any belief system;
- creates anger towards God;
- questions the meaning of suffering;
- verbalizes the inner conflict about beliefs;
- verbalizes the concern about relationships with deity;
- questions the meaning of our own existence;

- prevents participation in usual religious practices;
- seeks spiritual assistance;
- questions moral or ethical implications of therapeutic regimen;
- humour becomes 'gallows humour';
- displaces anger towards religious representatives;
- gives nightmares of sleep disturbance;
- alters the behaviour or mood evidenced by anger, crying, withdrawal, preoccupation, anxiety, hostility or apathy.

This notion of spiritual distress appears to suggest that it is something that may occur in those who have previously held religious beliefs and who are now questioning them. It is suggested here that the notion of spiritual distress may be better conceptualized as a concern with ultimate things and with meaning. In this way it is quite possible to argue that atheists and agnostics are just as capable of experiencing spiritual distress as those who have, or who have had, religious convictions (Burnard, 1988). Spiritual distress, in these terms, is characterized more than anything else by a profound sense of *meaninglessness*.

This sense of meaninglessness is well described in the literature. Sartre's hero (or anti-hero) in *Nausea* experiences that feeling. He finds himself caught up in the world but not really part of it. He notices himself observing others but not being moved by them. In fact he is rarely moved by anything. Instead he experiences a profound sense of isolation and distaste for life. Such a position is one that Hesse's character, Harry Haller, in *Steppenwolf* is familiar with. Aware of a 'darker' side to his personality, Haller also feels himself to be an observer of life rather than a participant in it.

Sometimes, such meaninglessness comes as a result of working in situations that are demanding of our emotions. The processes of caring for others, of listening to other people's problems and of having to be altruistic all take their toll. We cannot expect to continue to give to others without at some point feeling a sense of being 'used up'. Unfortunately, as we have noted, the health professionals are not, generally, very good at supporting each other. Thus it is quite possible to be in a caring role and have continual demands made on one's time and resources without anyone else attempting to life the load. In time, it is possible to reach a state of meaninglessness through sheer emotional (and possibly, spiritual) exhaustion.

VALUES CLARIFICATION

One approach to coming to terms with meaning is through the process known as values clarification. If we are clear about what we value and feel to be important, we can cope more easily with many of the dilemmas that face us in our personal and also in our professional lives. Such clarification can arise out of discussion and dispute with friends and colleagues. It can also be aided by conscious consideration of a number of difficult ethical issues and matters of principle. The Appendix on page 169 offers a Values Clarification Questionnaire. It may be filled in as an exercise in trying to sort out your own value system. It may also be used in a group or workshop context as the basis for discussion and argument. If we can be clear about what we believe and why we hold those beliefs, we may be less tempted to ignore or dispute the belief and value systems of others. Arguably, the health professions are not the place for evangelizing or proselytizing for a particular set of values or beliefs. We need to be aware of our own beliefs and values and must accept those of others.

Berne (1972) suggested that people tend to adopt certain life positions in relation to others. In this simple, economical way of considering life values and attitudes towards others, Berne suggests four possible life positions:

- I'm OK – you're OK.
- I'm OK – you're not OK.
- I'm not OK – you're not OK.
- I'm not OK – you're OK.

The people who develop the 'I'm OK – you're OK' position are essentially positive about themselves and about others. In being clear about their own values and themselves, they are able to accept the values and differences of other people. They are positive about themselves and about others.

The people who adopt the 'I'm OK – you're not OK' position are positive about their own values but are highly critical of others. Sometimes this is because they distrust or are uncertain of their own values. Sometimes it is because they hold their own values so dogmatically that they find it impossible to believe that other values can be held. Such people can appear arrogant and distant in their relationships with others.

The people who adopt the 'I'm not OK – you're not OK'

position doubt their own values and those of others. Essentially, they take a fairly dim view of themselves and of other people. This negative view of life tends to be self-reinforcing. The more these people look for weaknesses in themselves and others in general, the more they find those weaknesses to be evident! For these people, relationships are doomed to failure because of the inherent weaknesses in all humanity.

Almost as distressing as the above life position is that of the people who adopt the 'I'm not OK – you're OK' position. These people feel that the rest of the world is superior. Everyone else manages and copes while they battle and fail.

The process of clarifying values can help to establish or re-establish the position of 'I'm OK – you're OK'. In the end, this position must be the best one for the health professionals to adopt both personally and professionally. The other life positions either tend to lead towards very painful lives or they cause the health professionals to develop a bitter and cynical view of their jobs and of their clients.

Berne's analysis of life positions is also a useful framework through which to consider how *clients* view their lives. Very often, people who seek out a health professional for help with problems in living or emotional difficulties are adopting the 'I'm not OK – you're OK' position in relation to that health professional. They have often adopted that position in relation to other people in their lives as well. Just acknowledging the style of life position that is being played out in the client–professional relationship can help in attempting to redress the balance. Berne's analysis offers a simple yet effective way of exploring relationships.

MEDITATION

Another approach to the question of meaning is through contemplation and thoughtfulness, via meditation. Clearly, all sorts of other approaches are possible, from pastoral counselling, through intensive psychotherapy to help from church workers. Discussion with friends is another approach to tackling these fundamental questions of meaning. It is also important to differentiate questions of meaning from clinical depression. The depressed person, after all, may exhibit some or all of the above characteristics. When clinical depression exists, it should be treated through one of the many psychological and pharmacological approaches available. Why, then, the recommendation of meditation?

In the end, questions of meaning involve what Kierkegaard called a 'leap of faith'. It seems unlikely that there will ever be factual, empirical evidence to help us untangle questions of meaning. In the end, we have to decide for ourselves. What we believe, what sustains us, can only come through inner conviction. That inner conviction cannot be given to us by another person, we can only experience it (or not experience it) for ourselves. In the normal flow of life we are constantly being caught up in the processes of thinking about our work, our families, our commitments and so on. We rarely have time to sit and quietly think through our beliefs or lack of them. If nothing else, meditation can offer a time of peace and quiet during or after which we may be able to apply ourselves to thinking about our own beliefs and meaning systems. A fortunate side effect of meditation, too, is what Benson (1975) called the 'relaxation response'. Thus we may not only begin to sort out our beliefs but we shall also be helped to relax in the process. In this sense, then, meditation offers a two-pronged approach to dealing with stress: (a) it can help us to relax and (b) it can help us, if we wish, to puzzle out some of our own solutions to ultimate questions.

Meditation has been used for centuries for mystical, religious and secular purposes. There are many excellent accounts of the history and theory behind various meditational practices (see, for example, Tart, 1969; Le Shan, 1974; Hewitt, 1977; Pearce, 1982; Bond, 1986). The following activities are simple and effective. They can be used to explore self-awareness or they can be used simply as a means of inducing relaxation. They can be used by the individual or by a small group. They are described as though they relate to the individual meditating alone. If they are used in a small group setting, it is advisable to find a room where people can be undisturbed and quiet. It is also probably better if the facilitator does not try too hard to invoke a 'mysterious' atmosphere.

Practical Methods of Coping with Stress in the Health Professions: 6

TREAT YOURSELF

Stressful periods are often also busy periods. At such times it is important to allow at least some time in each week that you devote to yourself. Use that time to do something quite different. Indulge yourself. Do something new. It is sometimes the case that we do not need to relax so much as needing to do something that both suits us and does not involve our doing things for others.

Simple calming techniques

Brande (1934) describes two simple techniques, related to meditation, which help to reduce tension. Both require practise but both are easy to carry out on your own or in the company of others.

The first method involves attempting to clear the mind of unwanted distractions. Close your eyes and concentrate on holding your mind quite steady but do not feel any urgency or tension about doing this. At first, you may only achieve this holding for a few moments. As you practise, however, it is possible to begin to calm the mind and to 'hold' it for longer periods. Initially, the 'roof-brain chatter' that Pearce (1982) describes will tend to crowd in and distract you. Roof-brain chatter is the whole stream of thoughts and ideas that tends to rush through our mind as soon as we start to reflect on that mind.

The second method that Brande describes involves the holding of a simple object that you can cup in your hand. Hold the object and attempt to confine your attention to it. If your thoughts start to wander, slowly bring them back to the object. Again, allow yourself to acknowledge and be distracted by roof-brain chatter, at first. As you become more used to the activity you will find it possible to concentrate on the object for longer periods.

These activities were suggested by Brande as methods for helping writers to improve their writing output. If you are engaged in writing projects you may want to use them in this way, although they are useful stress reduction agents in their own right.

Meditation Technique 1

NOTICING THE BREATHS

1. Sit motionless, comfortably and with the eyes closed.
2. Breathe quietly and gently. Breathe in through the nostrils and out through the mouth.

3. Let your attention focus on your breathing.
4. Begin to count your breaths, from one to ten. One is the whole cycle of an inhalation and an exhalation. Two is the next complete cycle.
5. When the breaths have been counted from one to ten, begin to count the next set from one to ten and so on.
6. If you are distracted or lose count, simply go back to the beginning and start again.

In the early stages of meditation, it is very easy to be distracted by what Pearce calls 'roof-brain' chatter (Pearce, 1982), the seemingly endless flow of thoughts and ideas that refuse to go away when we sit down to meditate. Meditation, like most things, take practise and commitment. Slowly, the roof-brain chatter dies away.

Meditation Technique 2

Lie on your back with your hands by your sides . . . stretch your legs out and have your feet about a foot apart . . . pay attention to your breathing . . . now let your breathing become gentle and relaxed . . . now I want you to experience your body growing in size . . . your head, your arms, your legs, your trunk . . . are all growing in size . . . experience that sense of growing and allow yourself to grow more . . . experience your growing until your head reaches the top of the ceiling . . . feel your vastness . . . and experience a feeling of calmness and equanimity . . . now continue to grow . . . your head goes up into the sky . . . until all the surrounding town and countryside is contained within you . . . you are continuing to grow . . . you grow larger still . . . feel your vastness . . . until your head is among the planets and you are sitting in the middle of the galaxy . . . the Earth is lying deep inside you . . . feel all this and experience the feeling of vastness . . . of awe . . . of calmness . . . sit in this universe . . . silent, huge, peaceful . . . continue to grow . . . until you contain all the galaxies . . . you are at one with everything . . . experience the vastness . . . let everything be as it is . . . the silence.

Now, very slowly, allow yourself to return . . . come down in size slowly . . . past the galaxy . . . down, slowly to the size of the Earth . . . now slowly to the surrounding countryside and towns and notice all that is around you . . . now continue to come down in size until you fill the room . . . slowly, gently . . . now return to your normal size . . . and just lie for a while and experience the sense of peace and relaxation . . . think of your experience . . . remain quiet and relaxed . . . take a couple of deep breaths . . . in your own time . . . slowly stretch . . . sit up gently . . . and open your eyes.

Meditation Technique 3

USING A MANTRA

A mantra is a particular word or phrase that is repeated over and over again as an aid to stilling and calming the mind. Many religious and mystical traditions use repetitious phrases as part of their rituals and sometimes the mantra is a sacred sound of expression. Examples of mantras drawn from various traditions are as follows:

- *om* (prounounced 'aum')   This is probably the best known of all mantras and the most widely used.
- *om namah shivaya*   This is a traditional Indian mantra and translates, roughly, as 'I honour my own self' or, more literally, 'I bow to Shiva'.
- *om mani padme hum*   This is usually translated as 'The Jewel in the Lotus'.
- *la ilaha illa llah*   This is a line from the Koran and means 'There is no God but Allah'.
- *kyrie eleison*   This is a Greek phrase, used widely in the Christian tradition.

The following phrases could be used as Christian mantras:

- Be still and know that I am God.
- Lord Jesus Christ, son of God, have mercy on me.

Stoll (1989), adapting the work of Benson (1984), offers a series of phrases that can be used in contemplative and meditative work. She divides these up according to various religions, as follows:

For Roman Catholic and other Christian traditions:

- Variations on the prayer: 'Our Father who art in heaven' or 'Hallowed by Thy name'.
- Phrases from the Hail Mary: 'Hail Mary, full of grace . . .'.
- A phrase from Mary's Magnificat, Luke 1:46–55: 'My soul magnifies the Lord'.

For Protestants:
- Psalm 23: 'The Lord is my shepherd'.
- Psalm 100: 'Make a joyful noise unto the Lord'.
- Jesus' teachings or words: 'My peace I give to you' (John 4:27) or 'Love one another' (John 15:12).

Other meaningful passages from the New Testament, such as 'The peace which passes all understanding' (Phil. 4:7) or 'We have the mind of Christ' (1 Cor. 2:16).

For Jewish people:
- The Hebrew word for *peace*: Shalom.
- The Hebrew word for *one*: Echod.
- Passages from the Old Testament such as 'You shall love your neighbour' (Lev. 19:18) or God said 'Let there be light' (Gen. 1:3).
- Phrases that conform to King David's practice of meditating on God's promises, precepts, law, works, wonders, name and decrees.

For Moslems:
- The word for God, 'Allah': 'The Lord is wondrous kind . . .'.
- Adahum 'One God', the words of the first Moslem who called the 'faithful' to prayer.

For Hindus and Buddhists:
- The Bhagavad-Gita, the Hindu Scriptures, says, 'Joy is inward'.
- Part of a favourite invocation of Hindu priests: 'Thou are everywhere' and 'Thou art without form'.
- Buddhist literature contains phrases like these: 'Life is a journey' and 'I surrender indifferently'.

Still others prefer single words or even meaningless sounds. Words and expressions that have been used as mantras include: peace; love; harmony; be here now; I am one.

FOCUSING

Related to meditation but also different to it, is the process known as focusing. This is a simple process of allowing the body and mind to relax and thus enabling a 'felt sense' of one's problems to emerge. The process allows for a natural process of problem solving to occur. The focusing approach outlined here is based on that described by Eugene Gendlin (Gendlin, 1981; Hales-Tooke, 1989).

1. Sit quietly and breathe deeply for while. Allow yourself to relax completely. Notice the thoughts and feelings that flood into your mind. Slowly, but without worrying too much, identify one.
2. Having identified each thought or feeling that comes drifting into your mind, find some way of 'packaging up' each of those thoughts and feelings. Some people find it easiest to imagine actually wrapping each issue up into a parcel. Others imagine putting each item into a box and sealing it with tape. However you do it, allow each thought or feeling to be packaged in some way. Then imagine those thoughts or feelings, in their packages, laid out in front of you. Notice, too, the sense of calmness that goes with having packaged up your thoughts and feelings in this way.
3. Now, in your mind, look around at those packages and notice which one of them is calling for attention. Sometimes there will be more than one but try to focus on the one that is *most* in need.
4. Now unpack that one particular issue and allow it some breathing space. Do not immediately put a name to it or rush to 'sort it out'. Instead, allow yourself to immerse yourself in that particular issue.
5. When you have spent some minutes immersing yourself in this way, ask yourself: 'What is the *feeling* that goes with this issue?' Don't rush to put a label on it: try one or two labels, tentatively at first. Allow the label to 'emerge' out of the issue. The feeling that emerges in this way can be described as the 'felt sense' of the issue or problem.
6. Once you have identified this 'felt sense' in this way, allow yourself to explore it for a while. What other feelings go with it? What other thoughts do you associate with it? And so on.

7. Once you have explored the felt sense in this way, ask yourself: What is the *nub of all this?* As you ask this, allow the real issue behind all your thoughts to emerge and to surface. Often, the nub or 'bottom line' is quite different an issue to the one that you started out with.
8. When you have identified the nub or crux of the issue, allow yourself to explore that a little. Then identify what it is you have to do next. Do not do this too hastily. Again, try out a number of solutions before you settle on what has to be done. Do not rush to make up your mind but rather let the next step emerge of its own accord. Once you have identified the next thing that you have to do, acknowledge to yourself that this is the end of the activity for the time being.
9. Allow yourself some more deep breaths. Relax quietly and then rouse yourself gently.

This approach to meditation and problem solving can be very useful when you are under stress and unable to discover what is worrying you. It is a method of allowing problems and solutions to surface of their own accord rather than one that forces the use of logical or systematic thinking. It is, perhaps, more intuitive than rational. It can also be used as a system for helping *others* to solve problems.

SUMMARY

We all need meaning to make sense of what we do. This chapter has discussed the problem of finding meaning. It has also suggested that meditation offers one approach to finding meaning. Various methods of meditation, including the use of mantras, have been described. As with the relaxation activities in the previous chapter, these methods may be used by the individual health professional or by a group. They can also be used with client groups.

7

Stress and assertiveness

I find it stressful trying to persuade some doctors that there
are other occupations in the world!

Nurse tutor

Aims of this chapter

This chapter explores:

● The nature of assertiveness
● Becoming assertive.

We all live and work with other people. In the health professions
we are also often called up to give ourselves to other people in
various ways. This can mean that our own needs come secondary
to the needs of others. On many occasions this is right and appropriate. On others, we give in to the demands of others simply
because we either do not have the skills to make our own needs
known or because we have become so used to giving in to others
that we have forgotten how to assert ourselves. Either way, the
net result over time is stress.

THE NATURE OF ASSERTIVENESS

We have noted that caring and working in organizations both take
their toll on the individual. Sometimes the person's *own* needs
become subsumed within the demands of the organization or
profession. One positive way of coping with stress in organizations

and in the caring profession is to become more assertive. Assertiveness is often confused with being aggressive; but there are important differences. Assertive people are those who can state clearly and calmly what they want to say, do not back down in the face of disagreement and are prepared to repeat what they have to say, if necessary. Woodcock and Francis (1982) identify the following barriers to assertiveness:

1. *Lack of practise*: You do not test your limits enough and discover whether you can be more assertive.
2. *Formative training*: Your early training by parents and others diminish your capacity to stand up for yourself.
3. *Being unclear*: You do not have clear standards and you are unsure of what you want.
4. *Fear of hostility*: You are afraid of anger or negative responses and you want to be considered reasonable.
5. *Undervaluing yourself*: You do not feel that you have the right to stand firm or demand correct and fair treatment.
6. *Poor presentation*: Your self-expression tends to be vague, unimpressive, confusing or emotional.

Given that most health professionals spend much of their time considering the needs of others, it seems likely that many overlook the personal needs identified within Woodcock and Francis' list of barriers to assertiveness. Part of the process of coping with stress is also the process of learning to identify and assert personal needs and wants.

A continuum may be drawn that accounts for a range of types of behaviour, ranging from the submissive to the aggressive, with assertive behaviour being the mid-point on such a continuum (Fig. 7.1).

BECOMING ASSERTIVE

Heron (1986) has argued that when we have to confront another person, we tend to feel anxiety at the prospect. As a result of that anxiety we tend to either 'pussyfoot' (and be submissive) or 'sledgehammer' (and be aggressive). So it is with being assertive. Most people, when learning how to assert themselves, experience anxiety and, as a result, tend to be either submissive or aggressive. Other people handle that anxiety by swinging all the way through

SUBMISSIVE APPROACH (Pussyfooting)	ASSERTIVE APPROACH	AGGRESSIVE APPROACH (Sledgehammering)
The person avoids conflict and confrontation by avoiding the topic in hand	The person is clear, calm and prepared to repeat what he or she has said.	The person is heavy-handed and makes a personal attack of the issue.

Figure 7.1 Three possible approaches to confrontation

the continuum. They start submissively, then develop a sort of confidence and rush into an aggressive attack on the other person. Some other people deal with their anxiety by starting an encounter very aggressively and quickly back off into submission. The level and calm approach of being assertive takes practise, nerve and confidence.

Stress in Health Care: a Case in Point   7

A group of nursing lecturers in a large college of health begin a series of lunchtime workshops to explore methods of coping with stress. Each lecturer agrees to run one of the lunchtime sessions. The workshops are run on an experiential learning basis and are aimed at introducing a range of practical methods of dealing with stress.

The first workshop consists of a discussion group in which stressors are discussed. In this first session, too, group members agree on the type of stress reduction methods that will be introduced.

The second workshop is focused on relaxation methods and participants are encouraged to try for themselves two muscle relaxation exercises. The third workshop offers three methods of meditation and proves to be the most difficult but most popular workshop. The fourth, focuses on time management and cognitive approaches to stress reduction.

The workshops prove popular and the lecturers agree to meet on a regular basis to discuss their own progress with their own chosen stress reduction methods. They also agree to run the workshops for interested students as an extra-mural course.

Confrontation

Consider the following examples of Heron's three types:

The pussyfooting approach

1. 'There's something I want to talk to you about . . . I don't really know how to put this . . . whatever you do, don't take offence at what I have to say . . .'
2. 'I don't expect you will like this but I think it is better that I say it than keep quiet about it . . . on the other hand, perhaps its better to say nothing.'
3. 'I know that you have an awful lot of work and I don't want to add to it. Perhaps I ought to discuss what I have in mind with someone else.'

The sledgehammer approach

1. 'What you do annoys me. If you had any feelings at all, you wouldn't get home so late . . . but that's typical of you.'
2. 'I give up with you. I bet you don't even know what I'm upset about . . .'
3. 'Everybody round here is busy. I don't know why you think you're so special. I want you to take on another caseload.'

The assertive approach

1. 'I would prefer it if you could get home a little earlier.'
2. 'I'm feeling angry at the moment and I want to discuss our relationship.'
3. 'I would like you to consider taking on Mrs Jones and her family'.

Posture

Notice, too, in your own behaviour and that of others, that *posture* and 'body language' often have much to do with the degree to which a statement is perceived by others as submissive, aggressive or assertive. These types of postures and body statements may be described using Heron's three approaches, thus:

The pussyfooting approach

- Hunched or rounded shoulders
- Failure to face the other person directly
- Eye contact averted
- Nervous smile
- Fiddling with hands
- Nervous gestures
- Voice low pitched and apologetic.

The sledgehammer approach

- Hands on hips or arms folded
- Very direct eye contact
- Angry expression
- Loud voice
- Voice threatening or angry
- Threatening or provocative hand gestures.

The assertive approach

- Face to face with the other person
- 'Comfortable' eye contact
- Facial expression that is 'congruent' with what is being said
- Voice clear and calm.

What is notable from these descriptions of three different approaches to confrontation is that the pussyfooting and sledge-hammer approaches can have *physical* as well as psychological effects. The person who frequently adopts one of these two approaches when dealing with others will often find that the experience is both physically and emotionally stressing. Becoming assertive is a potent method of learning to cope with all aspects of personal stress. It can also help to overcome *organizational* stress in that the assertive person is rather more likely to express his or her own needs and wants and is more likely to be heard.

Assertiveness in practice

Examples of how assertiveness can be useful include the following situations:

- when used to express the idea that a person is being asked to do too much by an employer;
- when used by a person who has never been able to express his or her wants and needs in a marriage;
- when used by a health professional, when facing bureaucratic processes in trying to get help for a client;
- in everyday situations in shops, offices, restaurants and other places where a stated service being offered is not actually being given;
- when used by a health professional who is attempting to modify the organizational structure of the workplace.

Arguably, the assertive approach to living is the much clearer one when dealing with other human beings. The submissive person often loses friends because they are seen as duplicitous, sycophantic or as a 'doormat'. On the other hand, the aggressive person is rarely popular, perhaps, simply, because most of us do not particularly like aggression. The assertive person is seen as an 'adult' who is able treat other people reasonably, without recourse to childish or loutish behaviour. Hargie, Saunders and Dickson (1987) summarize the functions of assertiveness when they suggest that the appropriate use of assertive interventions can help individuals to:

1. ensure that their personal rights are not violated;
2. withstand unreasonable requests from others;
3. make reasonable requests of others;
4. deal effectively with unreasonable refusals from others;
5. recognize the personal rights of others;
6. change the behaviour of others towards them;
7. avoid unnecessary aggressive conflicts;
8. confidently and openly communicate their position on any issue.

All of these functions can enable people to reduce their stress levels in interpersonal communication. Much has been written about the topic of assertiveness and the reader is referred to the recommended reading list at the end of this volume.

Alberti and Emmons (1982) identify four major elements in assertive behaviour:

1. *Intent* The assertive person does not intend to be hurtful to others by stating his or her own needs and wants.
2. *Behaviour* Behaviour classified as assertive would be evaluated by an 'objective observer' as honest, direct, expressive and non-destructive of others.
3. *Effects* Behaviour classified as assertive has the affect on the other of a direct and non-destructive message by which that person would not be hurt.
4. *Socio-cultural context* Behaviour classified as assertive is appropriate to the environment and culture in which it is demonstrated and may not necessarily be considered 'assertive' in a different socio-cultural environment.

Thus Alberti and Emmons invoke some ethical dimensions to the issue of assertiveness. They are suggesting that, used correctly, assertive behaviour is not intended to hurt the other person, should not be perceived as being hurtful and that assertive behaviour is dependent upon culture and context. They further suggest that assertive behaviour can be broken down into at least the following components:

- *Eye contact* The assertive person is able to maintain eye contact with another person to an appropriate degree.
- *Body posture* The degree of assertiveness that we use is illustrated through our posture, the way in which we stand in relation to another person and the degree to which we face the other person squarely and equally.
- *Distance* There seems to be a relationship between the distance we put between ourselves and another person and the degree of comfort and equality we feel with that person. If we feel overpowered by the other person's presence, we shall tend to stand further away from them than we would do if we felt equal to them. Proximity in relation to others is culturally dependent but, in a commonsense way, we can soon establish the degree to which we, as individuals, tend to stand away from others or feel comfortable near to them.
- *Gestures* Alberti and Emmons suggest that appropriate use of hand and arm gestures can add emphasis, openness and warmth to a message and can thus emphasize the assertive approach.

Lack of appropriate hand and arm gestures can suggest lack of self-confidence and lack of spontaneity.

- *Facial expression/tone of voice* It is important that assertive people are congruent in their use of facial expression (Bandler and Grinder, 1975). Congruence is said to occur when what a person says is accompanied by an appropriate tone of voice and by appropriate facial expressions. People who are incongruent may be perceived as unassertive. An example of this is the person who says he or she is angry but smiles while saying it: the result is a mixed and confusing communication.
- *Fluency* People are likely to be perceived as assertive if they are fluent and smooth in the use of their voice. This may mean that those who frequently punctuate their conversation with 'ums' and 'ers' are perceived as less than assertive.
- *Timing* Assertive people are likely to be able to pay attention to their 'end' of a conversation. They will not excessively interrupt the other person, nor will they be prone to leaving long silences between utterances.
- *Listening* Assertive people are likely to be good listeners. Those who listen effectively not only have more confidence in their ability to maintain a conversation, but also illustrate their interest in the other person. Being assertive should not be confused with being self-centred.
- *Content* Finally, it is important that what is said is appropriate to the social and cultural situation in which a conversation is taking place. Any English person who has been to America will know about the unnerving silence that is likely to descend on a conversation if such words as 'fag' or 'lavatory' are used in certain settings! So will the person who uses slang or swear words in inappropriate situations. It is important, in being perceived as assertive, that a person learns to use appropriate words and phrases.

A paradox emerges from all these dimensions of assertive behaviour. Assertive people must also be genuine in their presentation of 'self'. If those individuals are too busy noticing their behaviour and verbal performance, they are likely to feel distinctly self-conscious and contrived. It would seem that assertiveness training, like other forms of interpersonal skills training, tends to go through three stages and an understanding of those stages can help to resolve that paradox.

Stage 1: The person is unaware of his or her behaviour and is also unaware of the possible changes that he or she may bring about in order to become more assertive.

Stage 2: The person begins to appreciate the various aspects of assertive behaviour, practises them and temporarily becomes clumsy and self-conscious in their use.

Stage 3: The person incorporates the new behaviours into his or her personal repertoire of behaviours and 'forgets' them, but is perceived as more assertive. The new behaviours have become a 'natural part of the person.

It is asserted that if behavioural change in interpersonal skills training is to become relatively permanent, the person must learn to live through the rather painful second stage of the above model. Once through it, the new skills become more effective as they are incorporated into that person's everyday presentation of self.

Practical Methods of Coping with Stress in the Health Professions: 7

BE MORE OPEN

Some people, when they are stressed, tend to become more introverted. Consider opening up and sharing yourself more with others. Some areas in which you might consider becoming more open include:

- *personal relationships,*
- *relationships with colleagues,*
- *relationships with clients,*
- *talking to seniors,*
- *seeking assessment from your boss*
- *admitting mistakes.*

Luft (1969) argued that there are two main keys to self-awareness: self-disclosure and feedback from others. Jourard (1971) suggested that self-disclosure was one of the prime factors in developing and sustaining satisfactory relationships.

LEARNING TO BE ASSERTIVE

In developing assertiveness in others, the trainer is clearly going to have to be able to role model an assertive behaviour. The starting point in this field, then, is personal development if it is required. This can be gained through attendance, initially, at an assertiveness training course and later through undertaking a 'training the trainers' course. There are an increasing number of colleges and extramural departments of universities which offer such courses and they are also often included in the list of topics offered as evening courses.

Once the trainer has developed some competence in being assertive, the following stages need to be followed in the organization of a successful training course for others.

Stage 1: A theory input which explains the nature of assertive behaviour, including its differentiation from submissive and aggressive behaviour.

Stage 2: A discussion of the participants' own assessment of their assertive skills or lack of them. This assessment phase may be enhanced by volunteers role-playing typical situations in which they find it difficult to be assertive.

Stage 3: Examples of assertive behaviour from which the participants may role-model. These may be offered in the form of short video film presentations, demonstrations by the facilitator with another facilitator, demonstrations by the facilitator with a participant in the workshop, or through demonstrations offered by skilled people invited into the workshop to demonstrate assertive behaviour. The last option is perhaps the least attractive as a performance that is too good can often lead to group participants feeling deskilled. It is easy for the less confident person to feel 'I could never do that'. For this reason, too, it is important that the facilitator running the workshop does not present himself or herself as being too assertive but allows some 'faults' to appear. A certain amount of lack of skill in the facilitator can be reassuring to course participants.

Stage 4: Selection, by participants, of situations that they would like to practise in order to become more confident in being assertive. Commonly requested situations, here, may include:

– responding assertively to a colleague;

- dealing with a client more assertively;
- returning faulty goods to shops or returning unsatisfactory food in a restaurant;
- not responding aggressively in a discussion;
- being able to speak in front of a group of people or deliver a short paper.

These situations can then be rehearsed using the slow role-play method. At each stage of the role-play, the participants are encouraged to reflect on their performances and adopt assertive behaviour if they have slipped into being either aggressive or submissive. Sometimes, this means replaying the role-play several times. Another learning aid, here, is the use of what may be called 'perverse role-play'. Here, the various situations are played out by the participants as *badly as possible*. In other words, the supposedly assertive person is anything but assertive and the 'client' behaves as badly as possible. It is often from these perverse situations that new learning about what *could* be done occurs.

Stage 5: Carrying the newly learned skills back into the 'real world'. Sometimes, the very act of having practised being assertive in the workshop is enough to encourage the person to practise being assertive away from the workshop. More frequently, however, there needs to be a follow-up day or a series of follow-up days in which progress, or lack of it, is discussed and further reinforcement of effective behaviour is offered.

Practical Methods of Coping with Stress in the Health Professions: 8

DEVELOP FLEXIBILITY

Stress can make us inflexible and resistant to change. Woodcock and Francis (1982) suggest that several skills are combined in the capacity to be flexible:

- *Accurately assessing situations.*
- *Listening to others.*
- *Continuously redefining the present.*
- *Not longing for 'the good old days'.*
- *Enjoying challenge.*
- *Admitting errors to oneself.*

HOW ASSERTIVE ARE YOU?

In this section you are invited to decide to what degree you are assertive in your relationships with others. First, consider the following areas and think about the degree to which you deal assertively (or otherwise) with other people:

1. At home
2. At work, with colleagues
3. At work, with clients or patients
4. With friends
5. In shops.

Now consider the following questions:

1. Which type of confrontation describes your style best?
(a) Pussyfooting.
(b) Sledgehammering.
(c) Confrontating.
2. What (if anything) stops you from being assertive?
    (a) Fear of rejection.
    (b) Feelings of inadequacy.
    (c) Feelings that other people are more important than you.
    (d) Fear of reprisal.
    (e) Other feelings.
3. What must you do to become more assertive?
4. What is likely to happen if you become more assertive?

This last question is important. If you are going to become more assertive, it is likely that other people will perceive you differently for a while. If you have had a tendency to be the 'pussyfooting' type, they are likely to see you as rather more pushy. If you have tended towards the 'sledgehammer' approach, they may see you as rather more subdued. Either way, other people are likely to be rather upset by your new 'presentation of self' and to want the 'old you' back. It is during this period that you need most courage and perseverance. The temptation to slip back to old ways is likely to be strong. If you want to deal with the world more on your own terms and to reduce the stress of always being subservant to the needs of others, such courage and perseverance pay off in the longer term.

SUMMARY

In order to care for others we must become clearer about our own needs and wants. If we want to reduce interpersonal stress we need assertiveness skills. The chapter has described the nature of assertiveness and offered a format for teaching and learning assertiveness.

8

Stress and its effects on you

The stresses I feel are made infinitely worse by the *fear of failure*.

Physiotherapist

Aims of this chapter

This chapter explores:

- Assessing **your** stress levels in your work
- Identifying your own coping mechanisms
- How other health professionals cope.

STRESS AND WORK

As we have noted previously, people who work in the health professions tend to become stressed by the nature of the job. Caring for others can be stressful in and of itself. In this section we shall discuss some practical methods of identifying those parts of your work that cause you stress. In the next section, a broader approach to stress and you is taken: you are invited to look at *all* the things that cause you stress.

For this exercise, consider the three squares in Fig. 8.1. They identify three aspects of the whole relationship between you and your work: the job, the environment and you. All three aspects are interrelated.

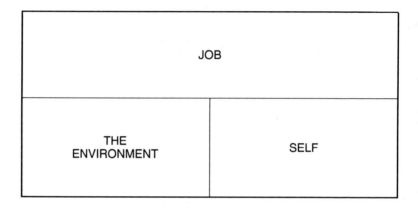

Figure 8.1 Three aspects of work related stress.

Take a sheet of paper and divide it into three. Now 'brainstorm' items under each of the three headings given in Fig. 8.1. Brainstorming is a way of creatively generating a range of ideas and thoughts. What you are required to do is to jot down anything associated with the heading (the job, the environment or you) that comes into your mind. Do not try to censor any particular items and do not leave anything out that seems, at this stage, irrelevant: everything counts. The following is an example of one social worker's brainstorming during this exercise.

The job

- Enjoyable but tough
- Hard work
- Doesn't necessarily stretch me.
- I can cope with it.
- I don't like the paperwork.
- I would like more management responsibility.
- Sometimes the clients get on my nerves.
- I'm not sure I can always cope with people who seem to be mentally ill.
- I think I could do more.
- I think I could be regraded.

The environment

- My office is too small.
- My office is drab.
- I can put up with the office because I'm not in it for very long during the day.
- I don't like the area in which I work.
- I don't like visiting the flats at night.
- I get anxious if I have too many visits to make.
- I don't get on with Mrs Davies.
- I don't like an number of my colleagues.
- I don't think all our caseloads are equal in terms of the work they involve.

Self

- I feel tense a lot of the time when I am working.
- I bring a lot of work home with me.
- I often find that I am thinking about work during the evenings.
- I don't have much of a social life.
- I don't like myself very much.
- I sometimes find myself counselling people about problems that are also my own but that I don't do very much about
- I need a holiday.
- I need a better relationship with my partner.
- I need to be more assertive

What is noticeable about this example of the brainstorming process is that the male social worker identified many of the stressors as being within *himself*. When you have done this part of the activity, ask yourself the following questions:

- Which aspect of my job seems to be causing me more stress than the other two (the job, the environment, you)?
- Which items in the list can I do something about and which items shall I have to put up with?
- What needs to be done to change any of these negative factors?
- Do any of the three lists of items indicate that I shall *have* to consider a change of job?

When you have considered these questions, draw yourself up a list of aims with regard to the issues in the three lists. Do not rush this part of the process and be realistic about what you can and cannot do and about what you can and cannot change. When you have drawn up this list of aims, copy them into your diary and use them as a checklist of things to work on. You may want to further subdivide the list into:

(a) immediate changes to be made;
(b) changes to work on;
(c) longer term considerations.

After considering all the changes that could be made and after realizing that he did not want to change jobs, the social worker who brainstormed the items above, drew up the following list:

Immediate changes

- Ring up local college of details of their assertiveness courses (this may help to put right a number of other issues).
- Discuss my work load with my boss.
- Invite friends round for meals for the next three Thursdays.
- Go to the library on the way home from work.

Changes to work on

- A more positive self-image (consider short workshops at the college that runs assertiveness courses)
- Keep up the contact with friends and make sure that I go to the cinema/concerts at least once a fortnight.
- Renegotiate my way of working with my colleagues.
- Reorganize the times I visit my clients.
- Pay off larger amounts on my credit card and then book a holiday for next year.

Longer term considerations

- More studying. Consider a part-time degree course starting next year. Find out about funding for this.

• Do I want to work in another area? This is not a short-term consideration but it may sensible in a couple of years' time.

LIFE STRESS ASSESSMENT

Another way of thinking about what causes you stress is to take more of a global look at your life. A well-known way of doing this is through the use of the Holmes–Rahe Social Readjustment Scale (Holmes and Rahe, 1967; Hanson, 1986; Fontana, 1989), Fig. 8.2. This is based on the premise that any changes in the routines of our lives cause stress. This is true of pleasant and welcome changes as well as difficult and unwanted ones.

Work on the social readjustment scale began in 1949 when Holmes and his colleagues carried out a study in which they asked over 5,000 people to report the life events that had occurred prior to the onset of their illnesses. Holmes drew up a list of the most common life events reported in the areas of the home, the family, work and the community over the ten years prior to illness. Holmes and Rahe (1967) suggested that such life events cause a change from the existing steady state of the person to a destabilized one.

It soon became evident that both positive and negative life events had an impact on the stability of the person. Holmes and Rahe asked almost 400 people to assign a quantitative score for the events on their list. Marriage was given an arbitrary value of 50. The other events were then ranked according to how individuals perceived them in terms of the amount of adaptation that the event required. Holmes found that of the people who scored a total of between 150 and 299 on the inventory, 53% experienced a health change. Of those with scores over 300, 80% reported significant health changes.

As we have noted, the scale assigns values to particular life events. You can use this scale to help you assess the degree to which you are stressed both in your work and in your life. The list is not complete. You may want to add your own stresses and stress values. You may also want to reflect on whether or not *you* would assign the values in the scale to *your* life events. As stress and stressors are such personal and idiosyncratic things, you may well decide that one factor is too highly rated or another has too low a value. Use the scale to get a general idea of your stress level: you do not need to tot up a score of your particular items.

Events	Scale of Impact
Death of spouse	100
Divorce	75
Marital separation	65
Jail term	63
Death of a close family member	63
Personal injury or illness	53
Marriage	50
Dismissal from work	47
Marital reconciliation	45
Retirement	45
Change in health of family member	44
Pregnancy	40
Sex difficulties	39
Gain of new family member	39
Business readjustment	39
Change of financial state	38
Death of close friend	37
Change to different line of work	36
Change in number of arguments with spouse	35
Major mortgage	31
Foreclosure of mortgage or loan	30
Change in responsibilities at work	39
Son or daughter leaving home	29
Trouble with in-laws	29
Outstanding personal achievement	28
Partner begins or stops work	26
Begin or end school	26
Change in living conditions	25
Revision of personal habits	24
Trouble with boss	23
Change in work hours or conditions	20
Change in residence	20
Change in schools	20
Change in recreation	19
Change in church activities	19
Change in social activities	18
Small mortgage or loan	17
Change in sleeping habits	16
Change in number of family get-togethers	15
Change in eating habits	15
Vacation	13
Christmas	12
Minor violations of the law	11

Figure 8.2 The Holmes–Rahe Social Readjustment Scale (reproduced with permission of Pergamon Press).

It is unlikely that the scale is as precise as this. On the other hand, you may want to add up your score on the inventory and decide the degree to which life events are affecting your well-being.

HOW DO YOU COPE WITH STRESS?

Another way of exploring your own stress and the things that cause you stress is the following exercise based on one suggested by Bond and Kilty (1983). First, note the three potential domains of stress identified in Fig. 8.3. The three domains that are identified are:

(a) causes of stress within myself;
(b) other people as stressors;
(b) causes of stress in the world at large.

Take three sheets of paper and head each up according to the three domains of stress. Next, brainstorm your thoughts about what causes **you** stress within the three. Follow the guidelines for brainstorming outlined in the previous activity. Consider the following sorts of issues under each of the headings:

CAUSES OF STRESS WITHIN MYSELF	
OTHER PEOPLE AS STRESSORS	CAUSES OF STRESS IN THE WORLD AT LARGE

Figure 8.3 Domains of potential stress.

Causes of stress within myself

- Do I like myself?
- Do I like the way I look?
- Do I take care of myself?
- Do I take notice of what others say about me?
- Do my moods affect my stress levels?
- Do I see myself as intelligent or not?
- Do I compare myself negatively with other people?
- What core values do I hold?
- What do I believe in?
- Do I eat properly?
- Do I look after my appearance?
- What do I most want to change about myself?

Other people as stressors

- Do other people upset me?
- Who, specifically?
- How do they do that?
- Are there particular sorts of people that I don't like?
- In what way are those sorts of people like me?
- How do I feel about my patients/clients?
- Are there particular people at work that irritate me?
- In what ways?

Causes of stress in the world at large

- Do political issues bother me?
- Which ones?
- What are my views about the ways other people live?
- What worries me about the way the world is at present?
- How do I feel about the work I do?

Now consider which of these issues stress you most and draw up a list of priorities for dealing with the most important issues. Identify, also, those issues that you *cannot* deal with. Once you have identified a list of priorities in this way, copy it into your diary and use it as a checklist for working through. You may want to classify those issues under the following three headings:

(a) immediate changes to be made;
(b) changes to work on;
(c) longer term considerations.

Work through your list, using as appropriate the activities suggested in this book. Remember, too, that you have to have the motivation to change: you cannot work on stress without changing *yourself*. The temptation is often to think that if other people round me change, or if I change certain incidental details about my life, everything else will fall into place! While the systematic approach to coping with stress may not suit everyone, the structure that is involved in identifying stressors in this way can help to clarify your thinking about what **you** need to do to change.

Practical Methods of Coping with Stress in the Health Professions: 9

'DOING' OR 'BEING'?

Many people in busy occupations spend a lot of time doing things. In the health professions this can mean that work is brought home, personal life is invaded with work and the health professional feels guilty if he or she is not doing something. Try concentrating for some time on being. Concentrate on who you are rather than on what you do. The fact that you take time to concentrate on your own needs rather than just on what you should be doing can enhance rather than detract from the care you give to others.

IDENTIFYING HOW YOU COPE WITH STRESS

Part of the process of coping with stress involves identifying the ways that *you* normally cope with stress. It is only when we have audited our own strategies that we can identify new coping mechanisms. The following activity offers one way of exploring how you have coped with stress until now.

On a sheet of paper brainstorm all the ways that you cope with stress, using the ground rules for brainstorming described above. Try to think of *all* of the things that you do to alleviate stress, both positive and negative. One nurse who undertook this exercise identified the following list:

119

- Smoke heavily.
- Worry!
- Leave difficult decisions.
- Remove myself from the stressful situation.
- Talk to my fieldwork teacher about my work.
- Bottle things up.
- Cry.
- Talk to friends.
- Talk to my boyfriend.
- Ignore what is happening and try to pretend that it isn't!
- Take a long bath.
- Go out for a drink.
- Argue with other people and become disagreeable with the patients.
- Write in my diary.

Once you have brainstormed all of the ways that you currently cope with stress, divide the list up into 'positive' and 'negative' methods of coping. Now ask yourself the following questions:

- Do the negative methods outweigh the positive?
- Do you tend to use the same sorts of ways of coping with stress all the time?
- Are there stress reduction methods that you could be using but do not?
- Do your stress coping methods interfere with your job as a health professional?
- In what ways?
- What methods of coping with stress do you *never* use?
- Why?

Again, this process of systematically identifying the methods you use to deal with stress can help you to think about *other* ways of coping. It is probably true that we get into fairly stereotyped channels of thinking and acting and rarely change our behaviour without considerable thought. A lot of our coping mechanisms seem to come into play without our thinking about them: they seem to be invoked at a 'unconscious' level. In order to change our strategies, we must first work consciously at changing. The activities described here can help to organize and systematize our approach.

120

Practical Methods of Coping with Stress in the Health Professions: 10

BEHAVIOURAL RELAXATION TRAINING

Schilling and Poppen (1983) describe a procedure they call Behavioural Relaxation Training. This includes the use of the following ten instructions for assessing relaxation:

1. *Breathing: relaxed.*
2. *Voice: quiet.*
3. *Body: no movement of the trunk.*
4. *Head: in midline, supported by recliner.*
5. *Eyes: closed with smooth eyelids.*
6. *Jaw: dropped, with lips parted.*
7. *Throat: no movement or swallowing.*
8. *Shoulders: sloped and even, no movement.*
9. *Hands: curled in resting posture.*
10. *Feet: pointed away from each other, forming a 90 degree angle.*

These ten criteria can be used as a personal checklist to assess the effectiveness of some of the relaxation exercises described in this book, when those exercises are carried out while lying down.

SUMMARY

We all experience and cope with stress in different ways. This chapter has offered a variety of methods of identifying your own stress levels and how you typically deal with stress. In the next chapter we consider ways of coping with stress through talking on a one-to-one basis or in a group.

9

Stress support systems for individuals

I experience stress every time I stand up in front of a
class . . .

Student teacher of physiotherapy

Aims of this chapter

This chapter explores:

* Counselling
* Co-counselling.

One very positive way of coping with stress is talking about it with
someone else. As we have noted elsewhere, feelings, thoughts and
problems that are confined tend to increase stress and tension.
On the other hand, releasing feelings, talking about thoughts and
discussing problems tends to lead to some resolution of stress.
Often, the informal talking through of difficulties with a friend or
partner is all that is required. Sometimes this is difficult: many
health professionals work in confidence and feel that they cannot
talk about their work-related problems at home or with friends.
  Alternatives to the more informal 'talking through' approaches
are the more structured approaches of counselling and co-counselling. Alternatively, support groups can be set up to allow for
the discussion of stressful issues in a supportive and conducive
atmosphere. This chapter explores the skills involved in counselling and co-counselling, and offers a description of the sorts of
events that happen in these activities. All of these approaches
involve fairly specific skills that can be described and learned, and

once learned individuals can often use such skills on themselves. People who learn co-counselling, for example, can soon use some of the skills and techniques involved to identify particular problems and attempt to find specific solutions. They can also learn to disassociate themselves from their stress, at least temporarily.

COUNSELLING

Counselling is available in various forms. On the one hand, there is the formal counselling that is offered by counselling agencies such as RELATE (The Marriage Guidance Council). On the other, there is informal counselling that takes place between friends or colleagues. The health professional who is stressed may choose the anonymity and confidentiality of the professional counsellors, or may feel more at home with friends. In either situation, the counselling skills discussed here will be of value. They will also be useful to the health professional who is attempting to help others who are stressed – whether colleagues or clients. Interestingly, too, the process of learning these skills can help us in counselling *ourselves*.

Counselling skills may be divided into two subgroups: (a) attending and listening and (b) counselling interventions. Attending and listening are by far the most important aspects of the counselling process. Often, the best counselling is that which simply involves the counsellor listening to the other person. Unfortunately, most of us feel that we are obliged to talk! Unfortunately, too, it is 'overtalking' by the counsellor that is least productive. If we can train ourselves to give our full attention and really listen to other people, we can do much to help them. First, we need to discriminate between the processes of *attending* and *listening*.

ATTENDING

Attending is the act of focusing, intentionallly, on the other person. It involves consciously making ourselves aware of what the other person is saying and of what he or she is trying to communicate to us. Figure 9.1 demonstrates three hypothetical zones of attention. The zones may help to clarify further this

OUTER EXPERIENCE	INNER EXPERIENCE
ZONE 1 'ATTENTION OUT' Attention is focused on the outside world and on the other person.	ZONE 2 'ATTENTION IN' Attention is focused on thoughts and feelings. ──────── ZONE 3 'FANTASY' Attention is focused on 'what might or should be the case' rather than on 'what is the case'.

Figure 9.1 Three possible zones of attention.

concept of attending and has implications for improving the quality of attention offered to the client.

Zone 1, in Fig. 9.1, represents the zone of having our attention fully focused 'outside' ourself and on the environment around us or, in the context of counselling, on the client. When we have our attention fully focused 'out' in this way, we are fully aware of the other person and are not distracted by our own thoughts and feelings.

There are some simple activities, borrowed from meditation practice, that can help to enhance our ability to offer this form of attention. Here is a particularly straightforward one. Stop reading this book for a moment and allow your attention to focus on some near object: it may be a clock, or a picture or a piece of furniture – anything. Focus your attention on the object and notice every aspect of it: its shape, its colour, its size and so forth. Continue to do this for at least one minute. Notice, as you do this, how your attention becomes fully absorbed by the object. You have focused your attention 'out'. Now discontinue your close observation. Notice what is going on in your mind. What are your thoughts and feelings at the moment? When you do this, you shift your attention to Zone 2: the 'internal' domain of thoughts and feelings. Now shift the focus of your attention out again and onto another object. Study every aspect of it for about a minute. Notice, as you do this, how it is possible to consciously and deliberately shift the focus of your attention in this way. You can will yourself to focus your attention outside yourself. Practise at this conscious process will improve your ability to focus attention fully outside yourself and onto the client.

Clearly, if we are to pay close attention to every aspect of the client, it is important to be able to move freely between Zones 1 and 2. In practice, what probably happens in a counselling session is that we spend some time in Zone 1, paying full attention to the client and then we shuttle back into Zone 2 and notice our reactions, feelings and beliefs about what they are saying, before we shift our attention out again. The important thing is that we learn to gain control over this process. It is no longer a haphazard, hit-and-miss affair but we can learn to focus attention with some precision. It is not until we train ourselves to consciously focus attention 'out' in this way that we can really notice what the other person is saying and doing.

Zone 3 in Fig. 9.1 involves fantasy: ideas and beliefs that we have that bear no direct relation to what is going on at the moment but concerns what we think or believe is going on. When we listen to a young male nurse, for example, it is quite possible to think and believe all sorts of things about him. We may, for instance, think 'I know what he's really trying to tell me. He's trying to say that he doesn't want to go back to work, only he won't admit it – even to himself!' When we engage in this sort of 'internal dialogue' we are working within the domain of fantasy. We cannot 'know' other things about people, unless we ask them, or as Epting (1984) puts it: 'If you want to know what another person is about, ask them, they might just tell you!' We often consider that we *do* know what other people think or feel, without checking with them first. If we do this, it is because we are focusing on the zone of fantasy: we are engaged in the processes of attribution or interpretation. The problem with these processes is that, if they are wrong, we can develop a very distorted image of other people! Our assumptions naturally lead us to other assumptions and if we begin to ask questions directly generated by those assumptions, our counselling will lack clarity and our client will end up very confused!

A useful rule, then, is that if we find ourselves within the domain of fantasy and we are 'inventing' things about the person in front of us, we stop and if necessary check those inventions with the client to test their validity. If the client confirms them, then we have intuitively picked up something about the client that, perhaps, we were not consciously or overtly being told. If, on the other hand, we are wrong, it is probably best to abandon the fantasy entirely. The fantasy, invention or assumption probably tells us more about our own mental make up than it does about that of our client! In fact, these 'wrong' assumptions can serve to help us gain more self-awareness. In noticing the wrong assumptions we make about others, we can reflect on what those assumptions tell us about ourselves.

Awareness of focus of attention and its shift between the three zones has implications for all aspects of counselling. The counsellor who is able to keep attention directed out for long periods is likely to be more observant and more accurate than the counsellor who is not. The counsellor who can discriminate between the zone of thinking and the zone of fantasy is less likely to jump to conclusions about his or her observations or to make value-judgements based on interpretation rather than on fact.

What is being suggested here is that we learn to focus directly on the other person (Zone 1) with occasional moves to the domain of our own thoughts and feelings (Zone 2) but that we learn, also, to attempt to avoid the domain of fantasy (Zone 3). It is almost as though we learn to meet a client as a 'blank slate': we know little about clients until they tell us who they are. To work in this way in counselling is, almost paradoxically, much more empathic. We learn, rapidly, not to presume things about other people but to listen to them and check any intuitions we may have about them.

Being able to focus on Zone 1 and have our attention focused out has other advantages. In focusing in this way, we can learn to maintain the 'therapeutic distance' referred to in a previous chapter. We can learn to distinguish clearly between the client's problems and our own. It is only when we become confused by having our attention focused partly on the client, partly on our own thoughts and feelings and partly on our fantasies and interpretations that we begin to get distracted about what the client is telling us and what we are 'saying to ourselves'. We easily confuse our own problems with those of the client.

Second, we can use the concept of the three domains of attention to develop self-awareness. By noticing the times when we have great difficulty in focusing attention 'out', we can learn to notice points of stress and difficulty in our own lives. Typically, we shall find it difficult to focus attention 'out' when we are tired, under pressure or emotionally distressed. The lack of attention that we experience can serve as a signal that we need to stop and take stock of our own life situation. Further, by allowing ourselves consciously to focus 'in' on Zones 2 and 3 – the process of introspection – we can examine our thoughts and feelings in order to understand ourselves further. Indeed, this process of self-exploration seems to be essential if we are to be able to offer another person sustained attention. If we constantly suppress problems we shall find ourselves distracted by what the client has to say. Typically, when the client begins to talk of a problem that is also a problem for us, we shall suddenly find our attention distracted to Zone 2, and shall find ourselves pondering our own problems and not those of the client! Regular self-examination can help us to clear away, at least temporarily, some of the more pressing personal problems that we experience. A case, perhaps, of 'counsellor, counsel thyself!'.

Such exploration can take be carried out either in isolation, in pairs or in groups. The skills exercises part of this book offers practical suggestions as to how such exploration can be developed. If done in isolation, meditative techniques can be of value. Often, however, the preference will be to conduct such exploration in pairs or in groups. In this way, we gain further insight through hearing other people's thoughts, feelings and observations and we can make useful comparisons between other people's experiences and our own. There are a variety of formats for running self-awareness groups, including sensitivity groups, encounter groups, group therapy and training groups. Such groups are often organized by colleges and extramural departments of universities, but they can also be formed on a 'do-it-yourself' basis. Ernst and Goodison (1981) offer some particularly useful guidelines for setting up, running and maintaining a self-help group for self-exploration. Such a group is useful as a means of developing self-awareness, as a peer support group for talking through counselling problems and also as a means of developing further counselling skills. Trying out new skills in a safe and trusting environment is often a better proposition than trying them out with real clients!

LISTENING

Listening is the process of 'hearing' the other person. This involves not only noting the things that they say, but also involves an entire range of other aspects of communication: tone of voice, use of catchphrases, expressions and so on. Given the wide range of methods in which one person tries to communicate with another, this is further evidence of the need to develop the ability to offer close and sustained attention, as outlined above. Linguistic aspects of speech refer to the actual words the clients use, to the phrases they choose and to the metaphors they use to convey how they are feeling. Attention to such metaphors is often useful as metaphorical language can often convey more than the conventional use of language (Cox, 1978b). Paralinguistics refers to all those aspects of speech that are not words. Thus, timing, volume, pitch, accent are all paralinguistic aspects of communication. Again, they can offer indicators, beyond the words they use, of how the other person is feeling. Again, however, we must be careful of making assumptions and slipping into Zone 3, the zone of fantasy. Paralinguistics can only offer us a possible clue to how the other person is feeling. It is important that we check the degree to which that clue matches the client's own perception of the way he or she feels.

Non-verbal aspects of communication refer to 'body language': the manner in which clients express themselves through the use of their bodies. Thus facial expression, use of gestures, body position and movement, proximity to the counsellor, touch in relation to the counsellor, all offer further clues about a client's internal status beyond the words that are used and can be 'listened' to by the attentive counsellor. Again, any assumptions that we make about what such body language 'means' need to be clarified with the client. There is a temptation to believe that body language can be 'read', as if we all used it in the same sort of way. This is, perhaps, encouraged by works such as *Manwatching* by Desmond Morris (1978). Reflection on the subject, however, will reveal that body language is dependent to a large degree on a wide number of variables: the context in which it occurs, the nature of the relationship, the individual's personal style and preference, the personality of the person 'using' the body language, and so on. It is safer, therefore, not to assume that we 'know' what another person is 'saying' with body language but, again, to treat it as a clue and to clarify with the client what he or she

128

means by its use. Thus it is preferable, in counselling, to merely bring to a client's attention the way he or she is sitting, or his or her facial expression, rather than to offer a dubious interpretation. Two examples may help here. In the first, the counsellor is offering an interpretation and an assumption:

'I notice from the way that you have your arms folded and from your frown that you are uncomfortable with discussing things at home'.

In the second example, the counsellor merely feeds back to the client what is observed and allows the client to clarify the situation:

'I notice that you have your arms folded and that you're frowning. What are you feeling at the moment?'

Use of 'minimal prompts'

While counsellors are listening to clients, it is important that they show that they are listening. An obvious aid to this is the use of what may be described as a 'minimal prompt' – the use of a head nod, a 'yes', or 'mm' and so on. All of these indicate that 'I am with you'. On the other hand, their overuse can be irritating to the client: particularly, perhaps, the thoughtless and repetitive nodding of the head – the 'dog in the back of the car' phenomenon! It is important that counsellors, at least initially are consciously aware of the use of minimal prompts and try to vary their repertoire. It is important to note, also, that such prompts are often not necessary. All the client needs is to be listened to and to appreciate that the counsellor is listening, without the need for further reinforcement of the fact.

Practical Methods of Coping with Stress in the Health Professions: 11

THE ALEXANDER TECHNIQUE

Stress can cause postural changes which in turn lead to tension and further stress. The Alexander technique (Alexander, 1969) offers a systematic method of learning to realign the position of the head in order to improve posture.

It also encourages the person to learn to make better 'use' of body movements. A simple experiment will illustrate the margin there is for improvement in this respect. The next time you switch on the television, note how you do it: pay attention to the full range of body movements you use. As you do this, you will probably become aware that you are using considerably more effort than you need to. The Alexander technique can help to train you in a more effective and efficient use of self. The technique is usually taught by individual practitioners but is sometimes the subject of evening classes at colleges and extramural departments of universities. It is acknowledged by most people in the field that it cannot be learned from a book.

Behavioural aspects of listening

The behaviour adopted by the counsellor when listening to a client, is also very important. Egan (1986) offers the acronym SOLER as a means of identifying and remembering the types of counsellor behaviour that encourage effective listening. The acronym is used as follows:

- Sit Squarely in relation to the client.
- Maintain an Open position.
- Lean slightly towards the client.
- Maintain reasonable Eye contact with the client.
- Relax!

First, the counsellor is encouraged to sit squarely in relation to the client. This can be understood both literally and metaphorically. In the USA and the UK it is generally acknowledged that one person listens to another more effectively if they are sitting opposite or nearly opposite each other, rather than next to each other. Sitting opposite allows the counsellor to see all aspects of communication, both paralinguistic and non-verbal, that might be missed if the counsellor sat next to the client. Second, the counsellor should consider adopting an open position in relation to the client. Again, this can be understood both literally and metaphorically. A 'closed' attitude is as much a block to effective counselling as is a closed body position. Crossed arms and legs, however, can convey a defensive feeling to the client and counselling is often more effective if the counsellor sits without crossing either. However, since many people feel more comfortable sitting with their legs crossed, perhaps some licence should be used here! What should be avoided is the position where the counsellor sits in a 'knotted' position with both arms and legs crossed.

It is helpful if the counsellor appreciates that he or she can lean towards the client. This can give encouragement and make the client feel more understood. If this does not seem immediately clear, next time you talk to someone, try leaning away from that person and note the result!

Eye contact with the client should be reasonably sustained, and a good rule of thumb is that the eye contact used by the counsellor should roughly match that used by the client. It is important, however, that the counsellor's eyes should be 'available' for the client; the counsellor is always prepared to maintain eye contact. On the other hand, it is important that the client does not feel stared at or intimidated by the counsellor's glare. Conscious use of eye contact can ensure that the client feels listened to and understood, but not uncomfortable.

The amount of eye contact the counsellor can make will depend on a number of factors, including the topic under discussion, the degree of 'comfortableness' the counsellor feels with the client, the degree to which the counsellor feels attracted to the client, the amount of eye contact the client makes, the nature and quality of the client's eye contact and so forth. If the counsellor continually finds the maintenance of eye contact difficult, it is perhaps useful to consider talking the issue over with a trusted colleague or with a peer support group, for eye contact is a vital channel of communication in most interpersonal encounters (Heron, 1970a).

Finally, it is important that counsellors feel relaxed while listening. This usually means that counsellors should refrain from 'rehearsing responses' mentally. It means that they give themselves up completely to the task of listening and trust themselves to make the appropriate response when necessary. This underlines the need to consider listening as the most important aspect of counselling. Everything else is secondary. Many people feel that they must have a ready response when engaged in conversation with another person. In counselling, however, the main focus of the conversation is the client. The counsellor's verbal responses, although important, must be secondary to what the client has to say. Thus all the counsellor need do is sit back and listen intently. Easily said, but not so easily done! The temptation to 'overtalk' is often great but can be subdued by experience and by a conscious decision not to make too many verbal interventions. All these behavioural considerations can help the listening process. In order to be effective, however, they need to be used consciously. The counsellor needs to pay attention to using them and choosing to use them. As we have noted, at first this conscious use of self will feel uncomfortable and unnatural. Practise makes it easier and with that practise comes the development of the counsellor's own style of working and behaving in the counselling relationship. No such style can develop if, first, the counsellor does not consciously consider the way he or she sits or listens.

In summary, it is possible to identify some of those things which act as blocks to effective listening and some aids to effective listening. No doubt the reader can add to both of these lists and such additions will be useful as they will be a reflection of your own strengths and limitations as a listener.

COUNSELLING INTERVENTIONS

Counselling interventions are all those things that a counsellor may say in the counselling relationship. The types of counselling interventions described here are those that can be called 'client-centred'.

The term 'client-centred', first used by Carl Rogers (1951), refers to the notion that it is the client who is best able to describe how to find the solutions to his or her problems in living. 'Client-centred' in this sense may be contrasted with the idea of 'counsellor-centred' or 'professional-centred', both of which may suggest that someone other than the client is the 'expert'. While this may be true when applied to certain concrete 'factual' problems – housing, surgery, legal, and so forth – it is difficult to see how it can apply to personal life issues. In such 'life' cases it is the client who can identify the problem and it is the client who, given time and space, can find a way through the problem to the solution.

Murgatroyd (1986) summarizes the client-centred position as follows:

- A person in need has come to you for help.
- In order to be helped they need to know that you have understood how they think and feel.
- They also need to know that, whatever your own feelings

about who or what they are or about what they have or have not done, you accept them as they are.

- You accept their right to decide their own lives for themselves.
- In the light of this knowledge about your acceptance and understanding of them they will begin to open themselves to the possibility of change and development.
- But if they feel that their association with you is conditional upon *them* changing, they may feel pressurized and reject your help.

The first issues identified by Murgatroyd – the fact of clients coming for help and needing to be understood and accepted – have been discussed in previous chapters. What we need to consider now are ways of helping those people to express themselves, to open themselves and thus to begin to change. It is worth noting, too, the almost paradoxical nature of Murgatroyd's last point: that if clients feel that their association with you is conditional upon their changing, they may reject your help. Thus we enter into a counselling relationship without even being desirous of the other person changing!

In a sense, this is an impossible state of affairs. If we did not hope for change, we presumably would not enter into the task of counselling in the first place! On another level, however, the point is very important. People change at their own rate and in their own time. The process cannot be rushed and we cannot will another person to change. Nor can we expect people to change and become more the sort of people we would like them to be. We must meet them on their own terms and observe change as they wish and will it to be (or not, as the case may be). This sort of counselling, then, is very altruistic. It demands of us that we make no demands of others.

Client-centred counselling is a process rather than a particular set of skills. It evolves through the relationship the counsellor has with the client and vice versa. In a sense, it is a period of growth for both parties, for each learns from the other. It also involves the exercise of restraint. The counsellor must show self-restrain from offering advice and from the temptation to 'put the client's life right'. The outcome of such counselling cannot be predicted nor can concrete goals be set (unless they are devised by the client, at his or her request). In essence, client-centred counselling involves an act of faith: a belief in the other person's ability to find solutions through the process of therapeutic conversation and through the act of being engaged in a close relationship with another human being.

Certain, basic client-centred skills may be identified, although, as we have noted, it is the total relationship that is important. Skills exercised in isolation amount to little: warmth, genuineness and positive regard must also be present. On the other hand, if basic skills are not considered, then the counselling process will probably be shapeless or it will degenerate into the counsellor becoming prescriptive. The skill of standing back and allowing the client to find his or her own way is a difficult one to learn. The following skills may help in the process:

• Questions
• Reflection
• Selective reflection
• Empathy building
• Checking for understanding

Each of these skills will now be considered in turn. Each skill can be learned. In order for that to happen, each must be tried and practised. There is a temptation to say 'I do that anyway!' when reading a description of some of these skills. The point is to notice the doing of them and to practise doing them better! While counselling often shares the characteristics of everyday conversation, if it is to progress beyond that it is important that some, if not all, of the following skills are used effectively, tactfully and skilfully.

Practical Methods of Coping with Stress in the Health Professions: 12

PREVENTING STRESS AT WORK

All aspects of work in the health professions can be potentially stressful. Atkinson (1988) suggests the following points for tackling job-related stress:

1. *Ensure a good person–job fit or make necessary adjustments.*
2. *Develop sensible, rational beliefs and attitudes to yourself, your performance and your job.*
3. *Change your behaviour in line with your new attitudes, including reviewing priorities.*

4. *Develop the right skills and behaviours to enable you to do your job to the best of your ability.*
5. *Develop a good social support network, both at work and with family and friends.*
6. *Keep as physically healthy as you can through sensible diet, sleep, exercise and so forth.*
7. *Learn to relax.*
8. *Learn to use leisure time sensibly.*

Questions

Closed questions

Two main types of questions may be identified in the client-centred approach: closed and open questions. A closed question is one that elicits a 'yes', 'no' or similar one-word answer. Or it is one in which the counsellor can anticipate an approximation of the answer. Examples of closed questions are as follows:

- What is your name?
- Where do you work?
- What causes you stress?
- Are you still depressed?

Too many closed questions can make the counselling relationship seem like an interrogation! They also inhibit the development of the client's version of the story and place the locus of responsibility in the relationship firmly with the client. Consider, for instance, the following exchange between manager and client:

Manager: Are you happier now . . . at work?
Health professional: Yes, I think I am.
Manager: Is that because you can talk more easily with your colleagues about your workload?
Health professional: I think so . . . we seem to get on better, generally.
Manager: And has your field work supervisor noticed the difference?
Health professional: Yes, she has.

In this conversation, made up only of closed questions, the

counsellor clearly 'leads' the conversation and also tends to try to influence the client towards accepting the idea of being 'happier now' at work and that the supervisor has 'noticed the difference'. One of the problems with this sort of questioning is that it gives little opportunity for the client to profoundly disagree with the counsellor. In the above exchange, for example, could the client easily have disagreed with the counsellor? It would seem not.

On the other hand, the closed question is useful in clarifying certain specific issues. For example, one may be used as follows:

> *Health professional:* It's not always easy at home. . . . the children always seem to be so noisy . . . and my wife finds it difficult to cope with them.
> *Manager:* How many children have you?
> *Health professional:* Three. They're all under ten and they're at the sort of age when they use up a lot of energy and make a lot of noise . . . It all gets on top of me and its beginning to affect my work.

Here, the closed question is fairly unobtrusive and serves to clarify the conversation. Notice, too, that once the question has been asked, the counsellor allows the client to continue to talk about the family, without further interruption.

Open questions

Open questions are those that do not elicit a particular answer: the counsellor cannot easily anticipate what an answer will 'look like'. Examples of open questions include:

– What did you do then?
– How did you feel when that happened?
– How are you feeling right now?
– What do you think will happen?

Open questions are ones that encourage the client to say more, to expand the story or to go deeper. An example of their use is as follows:

Supervisor: What is happening at home at the moment?

Student: Things are going quite well. Everyone's much more settled now and my son's found himself a job. He's been out of work for a long time.

Supervisor: How have you felt about that?

Student: It's upset me a lot . . . It seemed wrong that I was working and he wasn't . . . he had to struggle for a long time . . . he wasn't happy at all.

Supervisor: And how are you feeling right now?

Student: Upset. . . . I'm still upset . . . I still feel that I didn't help him enough.

In this conversation, the counsellor uses only open questions and the client expands on personal thoughts and feelings. More importantly, perhaps, the above example illustrates the counsellor 'following' the client and noting paralinguistic and non-verbal cues. In this way, the counsellor is able to help the client to focus more on what is happening in the present.

Open questions are generally preferable, in counselling, to closed ones. They encourage longer, more expansive answers and are rather more free of value judgements and interpretation than are closed questions. All the same, the counsellor has to monitor the 'slope' of intervention when using open questions. It is easy, for example, to become intrusive by asking, too quickly, questions that are too piercing. As with all counselling interventions, the timing of the use of questions is vital.

When to use questions

Questions can be used in the counselling relationships for a variety of purposes. The main ones include:

- For further information: e.g. 'How many children have you got?', 'What sort of work were you doing before you retired?'.
- To clarify: e.g. 'I'm sorry, did you say you are to move or did you say you're not sure?'; 'What did you say then?'.
- Exploration: e.g. 'What else happened?', 'How did you feel then?'.
- Encouraging client-talk: e.g. 'Can you say more about that?', 'What are your feelings about that?'.

Other sorts of questions

There are other ways of classifying questions, and some to be avoided. Examples include:

LEADING QUESTIONS

These are questions that contain an assumption that places the client in an untenable position. The classic example of a leading question is: 'Have you stopped beating your wife?'! Clearly, however the question is answered, the client is in the wrong! Other examples of leading questions are:

– Is it stress that's making your work so difficult?
– Are your family upset by your behaviour?
– Do you think that you may be hiding something . . . even from yourself?

The latter, pseudo-analytical questions, are particularly awkward. What could the answers possibly be?

VALUE-LADEN QUESTIONS

Questions such as 'Does your homosexuality make you feel guilty?' not only pose a moral question but guarantee that the client experiences difficulty in giving an answer!

'WHY' QUESTIONS

These are difficult in a counselling conversation on at least the following counts:

(a) they tend to sound confrontational;
(b) they encourage people to offer you *theories* about how they feel rather than offering you a discussion of *how they are feeling;*
(c) they can be moralistic in tone.

CONFRONTING QUESTIONS

Examples of these may include: 'Can you give me an example of when that happened?' and 'Do you still love your wife?'. Confrontation in counselling is quite appropriate once the relationship has fully developed but needs to be used skilfully and appropriately. It is easy for apparent 'confrontation' to degenerate in moralizing. Heron (1986) and Schulman (1982) offer useful approaches to effective confrontation in counselling.

Funnelling

Funnelling (Kahn and Cannell, 1957) refers to the use of questions to guide the conversation from the general to the specific. Thus, the conversation starts with broad, open questions and, slowly, more specific questions are used to focus the discussion. An example of the use of funnelling is as follows:

Manager: You seem upset at the moment, what's happening?
Social worker: Its home . . . things aren't working out.
Manager: What's happening at home?
Social worker: I'm always falling out with Donna and the children.
Manager: What does Donna feel about what's happening?
Social worker: She's angry with me.
Manager: About something in particular?
Social worker: Yes, about the way I talk to Jason, my son.
Manager: What is the problem with Jason?

In this way, the conversation becomes directed and focused . . . and this may pose a problem. If the counsellor does use funnelling in this way, it is arguable that the counselling conversation is no longer client-centred but counsellor-directed. Perhaps, in many situations – particularly where shortage of time is an issue – a combination of *following* and *leading* may be appropriate. 'Following' refers to the counsellor taking the lead from the client and exploring the avenues the counsellor wants to explore. 'Leading' refers to the counsellor taking a more active role and pursuing certain issues that are felt to be important. If in doubt, however, the 'following' approach is probably preferable as it keeps the locus of control in the counselling relationship firmly with the client.

Reflection

Reflection (or 'echoing') is the process of reflecting back the last few words, or a paraphrase of the last few words, that the client has used in order to encourage him or her to say more. It is as though the counsellor is echoing the client's thoughts and as though that echo serves as a prompt. It is important that the reflection does not turn into a question and this is best achieved by the counsellor making the repetition in much the same tone of voice as the client used. An example of the use of reflection is as follows:

> *Tutor:* We had lived in the South for a number of years. Then we moved and I suppose that's when things started to go wrong.
> *Senior tutor:* Things started to go wrong . . .
> *Tutor:* Well, we never really settled down. My wife missed her friends and I suppose I did really . . . though neither of us said anything.
> *Senior tutor:* Neither of you said that you missed your friends . . .
> *Tutor:* We both tried to protect each other, really. I suppose if either of us had said anything, we would have felt that we were letting the other one down.

In this example, the reflections are unobtrusive and unnoticed by the client. They serve to help the tutor to say more, to develop his story. Used skilfully and with good timing, reflection can be an important method of helping the client. On the other hand, if it is over-used or used clumsily it can appear stilted and is very noticeable. Unfortunately, it is an intervention that takes some practise and one that many people expect to learn on counselling courses. As a result, when people return from counselling courses, their friends and relatives are often waiting for them to use the technique and may comment on the fact! This should not be a deterrent as the method remains useful and therapeutic.

Selective reflection

Selective reflection refers to the method of repeating back to the client a part of something that was said which was emphasized in some way or which seemed to be emotionally charged. Thus selective reflection draws from the middle of the client's utterance and not from the end. An example of the use of selective reflection is as follows:

> *Nurse:* We had just got married. I was very young and I thought things would work out OK. We started buying our own house. My wife hated the place! It was important, though . . . we had to start somewhere.
> *Senior nurse:* Your wife hated the house . . .
> *Nurse:* She thought it was the worst place she'd lived in! She reckoned that she would only live there for a year at the most and we ended up being there for five years!

The use of selective reflection allowed the client in this example to develop further an almost throwaway remark. Often, these 'asides' are the substance of very important feelings and the counsellor can often help in the release of some of these feelings by using selective reflection to focus on them. Clearly concentration is important, in order to note the points on which to selectively reflect. Also, the counselling relationship is a flowing, evolving conversation which tends to be 'seamless'. Thus, it is no reason to store up a point which the counsellor feels would be useful to selectively reflect! By the time a break comes in the conversation, the item will probably be irrelevant! This points, again, to the need to develop 'free floating attention': the ability to allow the ebb and flow of the conversation to go where the counsellor takes it and for the counsellor to trust his or her own ability to choose an appropriate intervention when a break occurs.

Practical Methods of Coping with Stress in the Health Professions: 13

TAKING A BALANCED APPROACH TO STRESS MANAGEMENT

Meg Bond (1986) suggests four basic approaches to the management of stress:

1. *Mental and physical distraction. Here, the person adopts various strategies to cope with stress through distraction.*
2. *Self-nurturance. Here, the person is more concerned with looking after herself as an approach to coping.*

3. *Confronting the problem. The approach, here is a rational, problem-solving one.*
4. *Emotional expression. Stress is dealt with by exploring the effect it has on feelings.*

A balanced approach to stress management may be one that draws on all four approaches. Consider your own strategies for coping with stress. Do you favour one approach rather than the others? If so, could you benefit from considering other methods?

Empathy building

This refers to the counsellor making statements to the client that indicate that he or she has understood the feeling that the client is experiencing. A certain intuitive ability is needed here, for often empathy building statements refer more to what is implied than to what is overtly said. An example of the use of empathy building statements is as follows:

> *Client:* People at work are the same. They're all tied up with their own friends and families . . . they don't have a lot of time for me . . . though they're friendly enough.
> *Counsellor:* You sound angry with them.
> *Client:* I suppose I am! Why don't they take a bit of time to ask me how I'm getting on? It wouldn't take much!
> *Counsellor:* It sounds as though you are saying that people haven't had time for you for a long time.
> *Client:* They haven't. My family didn't bother much . . . I mean, they looked as though they did . . . but they didn't really.

The empathy building statements, used here, are ones that read between the lines. Now, sometimes such reading between the lines can be completely wrong and the empathy building statement is rejected by the client. It is important, when this happens, for the counsellor to drop the approach altogether and to pay more attention to listening. Inaccurate empathy building statements often indicate an overwillingness on the part of the counsellor to become 'involved' with the client's perceptual world – at the expense of accurate empathy! Used skilfully, however, they help the client to disclose further and indicate to the client that he or she is understood.

Checking for understanding

Checking for understanding involves either (a) asking the client if you have understood him or her correctly or (b) occasionally summarizing the conversation in order to clarify what has been said. The first type of check is useful when the client quickly covers a lot of topics and seems to be 'thinking aloud'. It can be used to further focus the conversation or as a means of ensuring that the client really stays with what he or she has said. The second type of check should be used sparingly or the counselling conversation can seem to be rather mechanical and studied. The following examples illustrate the two uses of checking for understanding.

Example (a)

> *Student:* I feel all over the place at the moment . . . things aren't quite right at work . . . money is still a problem and I don't seem to be talking to anyone . . . I'm not sure about work . . . sometimes I feel like packing it in . . . at other times I think I'm doing OK.
>
> *Manager:* Let me just clarify . . . you're saying things are generally a problem at the moment and you've thought about leaving work?
>
> *Student:* Yes . . . I don't think I will stop work but if I can get to talk it over with my boss, I think I will feel easier about it.

Example (b)

> *Manager:* Let me see if I can just sum up what we've talked about this afternoon. We talked of the financial problems and the question of talking to the bank manager. You suggested that you may ask him for a loan. Then you went on to say how you felt you could organize your finances better in the future.

Student: Yes, I think that covers most things.

Some counsellers prefer to use the second type of check at the end of each counselling session and this may help to clarify things before the client leaves. On the other hand, there is much to be said for not 'tidying up' the end of the session in this way. If the loose ends are left, the client continues to think about all the issues that have been discussed, as he or she walks away from the session. If everything is summarized too neatly, the client may feel that the problems can be 'closed down' for some time or, even worse, that they have been 'solved'! Personal problems are rarely simple enough to be summarized in a few words and the use of checking at the end of a session should be used sparingly.

Summary

These, then, are particular skills that encourage self-direction on the part of the client and can be learned and used by the counsellor. They form the basis of all good counselling and can always be returned to as a primary way of working with the client in the counselling relationship.

Practical Methods of Coping with Stress in the Health Professions: 14

PARADOXICAL INTENTION

Sometimes, when we try to relax, this is just the thing we cannot do! Instead, it is helpful to tell yourself to become MORE stressed! Often, this method allows you, paradoxically, to relax. The fact that you give yourself permission to be the way you are also allows you to change. This method can also be used to help other people who are stressed or tense. Instead of imploring them to relax, the suggest is to become more tense.

CO-COUNSELLING

Co-counselling is a two-way process in which two people take turns to spend time as 'counsellor' and 'client'. The client takes time to verbalize and talk through issues and problems from everyday life, while the counsellor gives complete attention. The counsellor in this relationship does not act in the traditional counselling manner – in other words, no advice is offered and no attempt is made to 'sort out' the client. In this self-directed approach, the client learns to examine his or her own problems and be a 'self-counsellor'. Each individual normally spends about one hour in the role of counsellor and one hour in the role of client. In this way, true interdependence is established. Neither part is wholly dependent upon the other. Responsibility is shared, though responsibility for working through problems remains firmly with the client. The counsellor may be invited to make interventions at the request of the client, according to a predetermined contract established between them.

Co-counselling can be used in a variety of ways. It can be a means of de-stressing for health professionals working in areas of high emotional involvement. The process of verbalizing pent-up feelings to another person in an understanding and confidential atmosphere can be very therapeutic. Co-counselling can also be used as a means of developing self-awareness through the process of exploring inner thoughts and feeling and particularly buried emotion. It can also be used as a means of practical problem solving, of talking out personal problems and making decisions about any aspects of the person's life.

Co-counselling developed under the influence of Harvey Jackins in the USA (Jackins, 1965, 1970) and John Heron in this country (Heron, 1978; Heron and Reason, 1982). It has made its mark within the field of experiential learning. David Potts (in Boud, 1981) has described its use as a learning tool in a university course and James Kilty (1983) has suggested the use of co-counselling in student nurse training. It can be of particular value as a self and peer support system for health professionals working in clinical environments that are particularly stressful: intensive care units, children's wards, oncology departments, hospices, psychiatric units and so forth.

Co-counselling training usually takes place through a forty-hour training course, during the course of one week, over two weekends or through a series of evening classes. Advanced co-counselling and co-counselling teacher training courses are also organized in colleges and extramural departments of universities.

Figure 9.2 is a simplified map of the theory behind co-counselling. This is necessarily a simple guide to the theory and the reader

1. People are potentially autonomous, self-directing, positive and able to exercise freedom of choice.

2. HOWEVER, people are subject to a variety of stresses , throughout life: early childhood experiences, partings, bereavement, difficulties in relationships, spiritual doubts and so forth.

3. Such stresses cause emotions (e.g. fear, anger, grief, embarrassment) to become 'bottled up'. This bottling up stops the person from functioning fully.

4. Through talking out and through emotional release (trembling, angry sounds, crying, laughter), those pent-up emotions may be released. Such release is therapeutic.

5. The effect of emotional release is that it generates insight and enables the person to think more clearly, to become less stressed, more autonomous and more able to take charge of his or her life. The person feels less 'acted upon' and more able to exercise choice, and can also be spontaneous, positive and life asserting.

6. Co-counselling training, through working in pairs, offers people training in:

   (a) listening to and giving attention to others;
   (b) reviewing and re-evaluating life experiences to date;
   (c) the release of pent-up emotion (catharsis);
   (d) handling other people's catharsis;
   (e) problem-solving and life-planning skills;
   (f) self-awareness;
   (g) stress reduction.

Figure 9.2 A simple map of the theory of co-counselling.

is directed to the recommended reading list at the end of the book for a more thorough explanation of what is involved.

The assumptions behind co-counselling are that people are potentially autonomous and able to exercise choice. Through the process of living, the individual experiences various types of stress which cause the blocking or repression of emotions. If those blocked emotions can be freed, then the person can once again be capable of making life-decisions and exercising freedom of choice. Co-counselling aims at enabling the individual to express that blocked feeling and thus become more able to control his or her life.

There are implications, here, for professional practice. As a general rule, we usually want to calm people down who are frightened, reassure those who are crying and stop people from expressing anger. Could we as health professionals be trained to *enable* people to express those emotions as a therapeutic human act? In the fields of health care practice the value of such an approach is perhaps clear: expressed emotion is presumably better than repressed emotion. Pre- and post-operative situations, before and after childbirth and following a bereavement are all situations that involve emotional experiences. Health professionals can be trained to help their patients to express those feelings freely rather than (a) prematurely stopping them or (b) feeling inadequate and unable to cope. Co-counselling offers one approach to coping with emotion. First, it enables the individual to experience his or her emotional feelings and second, it trains people to handle other people's emotional release.

Co-counselling is a clear example of experiential learning in that it asks the individual to review past and present experience and to reconstruct his or her understanding in the light of the discoveries made. The co-counselling format is simple and can readily be adapted to a variety of learning situations in health professional education.

The co-counselling format can be modified in various ways. The simple pairs method can be used as an introductory activity at the start of a learning session. The group is divided into pairs and one person in each pair talks to the other about whatever is at the forefront of his or her mind. The partner listens but does not comment. After five minutes, the roles are reversed and the 'listener' becomes the 'talker' and vice versa. The pairs format can also be used to explore *particular* issues, e.g. the role of interpersonal skills training in health professional education – any topic that is relevant to the subject under discussion. The format offers an economical and simple method of identifying a wide range of views, thoughts, attitudes and beliefs. It also honours the *student's* views and is not heavily teacher-centred as are more traditional methods of teaching and learning.

SUMMARY

This chapter has explored the 'talking' approach to coping with stress, through counselling or co-counselling. These two approaches have been described and the skills involved in them identified. In the final chapter, group support and supervision are examined.

10

Group support and supervision

I find it helpful to talk things through with one or two people
I feel I can be very frank and honest with; on other occasions
I just talk about it to anybody . . .

Lecturer

Aims of this chapter

This chapter explores:

- Support groups
- Supervision

In Chapter 9 we saw how one-to-one relationships can help in the
process of coping with stress. This chapter examines how group
settings can also help. Groups are economical of time, allow the
sharing of various points of view and are a means of developing
solidarity within an organization.

SUPPORT GROUPS

A positive way of learning to cope with stress is through the
support group. Such a group may meet on a weekly basis or
may be a 'one off' workshop which enables group participants to
explore a range of issues relating to stress, including causes of
stress, ways of coping with stress and long-term strategies. Perhaps
the easiest way of understanding how such a workshop may be
organized is through a description of one.

AN EXAMPLE OF A WORKSHOP ON STRESS MANAGEMENT

It is useful to have some understanding of what a workshop on stress 'feels' like and how such a workshop can be run. What follows is a description of the activities in a one-day workshop. It makes extensive use of the principles of experiential learning (Weil and McGill, 1989) and adult learning theory (Knowles, 1984; Knowles and Associates, 1985) and acknowledges some of the problems that may arise in this sort of workshop.

Description

The workshop is attended by eighteen health professionals from various disciplines including social work, nursing, occupational therapy and physiotherapy. The workshop is led by the author and takes place in a large room in a local higher education college. The group members are seated in a circle. Beside the facilitator is a large flip-chart pad on an easel. The workshop starts promptly at 9.00 am.

The facilitator makes a personal introduction and invites members of the group to introduce themselves by stating:

(a) their name,
(b) their occupation,
(c) three other things about themselves.

These three headings are revealed on a pre-prepared flip-chart sheet. The sheet with the headings is covered by a top sheet, which is turned over by the facilitator as the group are invited to introduce themselves.

Each member of the group then makes a personal introduction. Some take their time over the task; others are faltering but are fairly hasty. When each person has been introduced, the facilitator suggests that each person repeats, slowly, the name by which he or she wishes to be known. Thus the facilitator states his first name. The round begins slowly but then speeds up and the facilitator urges the group to take time over the undertaking so that each person's name is heard by other members. This round is then followed by another slow name round. Group members are then invited to check the names of those people they are still unsure of. The facilitator checks one person's name, and others follow suit. The ice has been broken and the group looks and feels more relaxed.

Basic principles of the workshop are then spelt out. These are the voluntary principle and the proposal clause. The facilitator also spells out, clearly, the timing of the workshop, giving times of coffee, tea and lunch breaks. After this, questions are invited from the group. The group is clearly thawing out and beginning to talk more freely. A couple of people ask about the nature of the group and whether or not it will consist of lectures from the facilitator or whether or not it will be an 'encounter group'. The facilitator explains that the day will be activity based and allow for participants to explore their own stress and stressors and examine some practical methods of dealing with stress. These questions lead naturally to the first exercise.

The exercise is one carried out in pairs. Each pair nominates one member A and one B. A then talks to B for ten minutes about 'how I react to stress'. After ten minutes, A and B change roles and B talks to A about his or her reactions to stress. The pair are asked to note that the exercise is not a conversation. One member is only required to listen while the other talks. The exercise is a type of thinking aloud.

After the exercise, which has been timed by the facilitator (who on this occasion has no partner, so does not take part in the exercise), the pairs are invited back into the group. They then discuss the exercise in terms of **process** and **content**. Process refers to how it felt to do the exercise. Content refers to what was talked about.

The discussion is prolonged and thus forms the 'reflective' aspect of the experiential learning cycle.

Some of the issues that emerge during the two aspects of the discussion are as follows: tension; boredom; loss of interest in life in general; loss of concentration; moodiness; disinterest in work; difficulty with relationships; panic/fear; difficulty with sex; anxiety; frustration; feeling of being overwhelmed; loss of sleep; fatigue; depression; crying; walking away from the situation; going off sick; being judgemental of others; angry spells; etc.

The facilitator then ask the group for its reactions to the results of the discussion. Theories and comments put forward by group members include:

'We all seem to experience stress differently.'

'Some aspects of stress are common to all of us.'
'I thought I was the only one who got worked up over nothing: it's a relief!'

The discussion brings the first hour and a half to a close and the group breaks for coffee, still discussing the issues involved. On resuming, after the break, the facilitator suggests that members divide into small groups of three and four and discuss some of the causes of stress, under three headings:

- How I cause myself stress.
- How other people cause me stress.
- Causes of stress within the world at large.

These headings are adapted from suggestions by Bond (1986). Each group is given a flip-chart sheet and a fibre-tipped pen and invited to elect a chairperson who writes down all the comments from the group. That chairperson does not edit out any suggestions but writes everything down. This is a typical brainstorming session. It is suggested that no filtering or dismissal of ideas takes place. In this way, the group develop freedom to think broadly and creatively. Some of the causes identified by group members are as follows:

How I cause myself stress

- By pushing myself too hard.
- By having too high expectations for myself.
- By worrying too much.
- By not being assertive.
- By allowing other people to walk all over me.
- By agreeing with everybody, even when I don't really!
- By thinking about sex too much.
- By not getting what I want/need.
- By suffering from loss of confidence/self doubt.
- By not thinking about my relationships with others.
- By not planning my work.
- By allowing myself to get depressed.
- By allowing others to decide what I should do.

How other people cause me stress

- By demanding too much of me.
- By not agreeing with me.
- By manipulating me.
- By putting pressure on me to succeed.
- By comparing me with other people (particularly at work).
- By not really knowing me.
- By getting aggressive with me.
- By belittling me.
- By being too bossy/authoritarian.
- By not communicating with me.
- By leaving me out in the cold.
- By not being honest with me.
- By being too easy with me.
- By doing things I don't like.
- By their anti-social habits (smoking, drinking, etc).

Causes of stress within the world at large

- Threat of nuclear war.
- Violence and bombings.
- Child abuse.
- 'Pressure', in general.
- Lack of purpose.
- Speed.
- Rise in the cost of living.
- Rise in the mortgage rate.
- Abuse of animals.
- Lack of housing.
- Lack of health care resources.
- Unemployment.
- The government.

This exercise, in groups, runs for twenty minutes after which time the facilitator invites group members to stick their charts on the wall and to examine other people's charts as they go up. After this, there is a discussion about the process as well as the content of the exercise.

The group is then invited to draw conclusions (or to theorize) on what has happened. Some responses, here, include:

153

'I mostly create my own stress!'
'I tend to believe that everyone is stressed for most of the time.'
'I'm surprised how quickly we have got to know each other here.'
'I found the discussion of sexuality embarrassing but useful.'

This exercise is the last of the morning. As a closing activity, each person in turn is asked to state, first of all, what he or she liked least about the morning. They are told that they need not qualify what they say but should feel free to say anything they like. After this round is completed, they are then encouraged to say what they liked most about the morning and, again, it is suggested that they do not need to justify or qualify what they say. The facilitator joins in both rounds. Some of the comments from group members are illustrated below:

'What I liked least about the morning':
- The initial embarrassment.
- Joining in with the pairs exercises, first thing.
- Discussion of embarrassing subjects!'
- I thought things were a bit slow to start with.

'What I liked most about the morning':
- Meeting new people.
- Comparing experience with other people.
- Realizing that other people feel the same as me!
- Pairing off.
- Being listened to but not judged.

Before breaking for lunch, the facilitator proposes a brief 'unfinished business' session. In this period of five minutes, group members are invited to say anything they like, either to other group members or to the facilitator, either positive or negative, that they may be thinking or feeling. The rationale behind this activity (and this is made explicit to the group) is to raise any 'hidden agendas' and to allow further self-disclosure. It also works on the principle that it is perhaps better that things are said rather than just thought. After an initial period of silence, one person says:

'I felt quite stirred up by the discussion this morning . . . I'm surprised how easily I get worked up.'

Another says:

'I'm a bit annoyed that you rushed me this morning (to the facilitator) and would have preferred more time to finish what I was saying!'

One member says to another:

'I enjoyed the pairs exercise with you this morning. I think we've got quite a bit in common!'

After the five-minute period, the group disperses and goes to lunch.

The afternoon session starts with a modified 'icebreaker'. All members are invited to say something about themselves that they are proud of. If may be something that they have achieved or a personal quality. As usual, the facilitator takes part in the round. The round seems to recreate an atmosphere in which group members can easily talk and self-disclose.

Following this, the group brainstorms methods of relieving stress. In this activity, the facilitator acts as scribe and records the suggestions of the group on a series of flip-chart sheets. Examples of some of the methods of stress relief that are identified by the group include the following: sleep; walking/cycling/exercise; massage; drinking alcohol; using tranquillizer in small doses; having a bath; eating; smoking; relaxation exercises; time management; taking sick leave; taking a holiday; meditation; yoga; having a good laugh/cry; counselling and co-counselling; change of activity; organization; discussion of relationships with the people involved; learning to be assertive; etc.

A discussion is then developed on the most common methods of stress relief: those that work and those that don't. As with the morning's session, there is some surprise and some relief that many people's experiences are similar.

The facilitator then asks the group to choose two methods from the list with which they are not particularly familiar and which they would like to try. After a brief discussion, they choose meditation and relaxation exercises. The facilitator then gives a brief theory input on the nature of relaxation exercises and on meditation. Theoretical information for such inputs can be found in Hewitt (1977), Naranjo and Ornstein (1971), Bond (1986) and Bond and Kilty (1983).

After this, the group undertakes a relaxation exercise. Once the relaxation activity has been undertaken, the group reforms and discusses the process of the activity. All, except one female member, have experienced complete relaxation. That person has, paradoxically, felt more tense through undertaking the activity and this is talked through with the person with the group's support. After the discussion of her feelings, the member feels considerably relieved and realizes that she gets most relief from stress through talking about the stressors in her life. This is useful not only for her but also for a number of other group members.

Following this discussion, the facilitator leads the group in a short meditation. The procedure for this is as follows:

1. Sit motionless, comfortably and with the eyes closed.
2. Breathe quietly and gently. Breathe in through the nostrils and out through the mouth.
3. Let your attention focus on your breathing.
4. Begin to count your breaths, from one to ten. One is the whole cycle of inhalation and exhalation. Two is the next complete cycle.
5. When the breaths have been counted from one to ten, begin counting the next ten and then the next, and so on.
6. If you are distracted or lose count, simply return to the beginning of the process and start again.

Following the 15-minute meditation, the group are again invited to discuss what happened. This time, all members find the activity relaxing and de-stressing and remarks are made about how they were physically and mentally able to relax. A member requests details of the two activities and the facilitator offers pre-prepared handouts. Many say that they wish to carry on using either the relaxation script or the meditation, at other times, away from the workshop.

After tea, there is an open-ended discussion about the day's events. Participants are invited to identify the high and low spots of the day and a closing round of 'least liked' and 'most liked' is carried out. The workshop finishes on a calm but interesting note and group members feel that it has been a worthwhile experience.

Practical Methods of Coping with Stress in the Health Professions: 15

HELP WITH WRITING

Nearly all health professionals have to write reports, letters, papers, articles and so on. Many people find the process of writing difficult and stressful. If we can learn to express ourselves clearly and easily in writing, we may save ourselves the stress of rewriting and editing. Robert Gunning (1968) offers ten principles of clear writing:

1. Keep sentences short.
2. Prefer the simple to the complex.
3. Prefer the familiar word.
4. Avoid unnecessary word.
5. Put action in your verbs.
6. Write like you talk.
7. Use terms your reader can picture.
8. Tie in with your reader's experience.
9. Make full use of variety.
10. Write to express not impress.

These principles can be used for any sort of writing from student projects to research reports and from papers for publications to day-to-day correspondence.

FACILITATING SUPPORT GROUPS AND STRESS WORKSHOPS

The above example of a workshop on stress describes one example of the workshop format. In that description, the term 'facilitator' is frequently used to describe the person who runs the workshop. It is useful to have some understanding of the options open to the facilitator of workshops of this sort or of groups that meet regularly to discuss stress and ways of coping with it.

John Heron (1989b) offers a six-fold model of facilitator styles (Fig. 10.1). The six aspects of facilitation are termed 'dimensions'.

The six dimensions of facilitator style may be used to make decisions about how any stress group or workshop may be run. It is not anticipated that all the dimensions will come into play in every group. Decisions about which dimension will be used during

1. THE PLANNING DIMENSION
2. THE MEANING DIMENSION
3. THE CONFRONTING DIMENSION
4. THE FEELING DIMENSION
5. THE STRUCTURING DIMENSION
6. THE VALUING DIMENSION

Figure 10.1 Six dimensions of facilitator style (Heron, 1989a)

the group will depend on the type of group being run, the aims of that group, the personality of the facilitator and the needs of the participants. The dimensions cover most aspects of setting up and running groups. The discussion here is an adapted version of Heron's model.

The planning dimension

This dimension is concerned with setting up the group. As group members should always know *why* they are in a particular group, the group facilitator needs to make certain decisions about how to identify the aims and objectives of the group. At least three options are available here:

1. The facilitator can decide upon the aims and objectives before setting up the group.
2. The facilitator can negotiate the aims and objectives with the group. In this case, the facilitator will decide some of those aims and objectives, and the group will decide others.
3. The facilitator can encourage the group to set its own aims and objectives. In this case, the facilitator simply supplies the 'title' or name for the group, and all other decisions about what the group is to achieve are made by the group.

The first option illustrates the traditional learning group approach. The facilitator – for example, a social worker – who uses this approach will have set aims and objectives for a particular lesson that have been planned in advance.

The second option illustrates the negotiated group approach. The facilitator – for example, an occupational therapist working as a group therapist – will meet the group for the first time and work with them to identify what that group can achieve in the time they meet together.

The third option illustrates the fully client-centred or student-centred approach to working with groups. Here, the facilitator – a health professional – does not anticipate the needs or wants of the group. Instead, the learning, therapy or discussion group is allowed to set its own agenda. Such an approach needs careful handling if it is not to degenerate into an aimless and sometimes pointless series of meetings.

Other aspects of the planning dimension include making decisions about the following issues:

- The number of group participants.
- The amount of time the group will spend together.
- Whether or not particular 'rules' will apply to the group.
- Whether or not group membership will remain the same throughout the life of the group (a closed group) or whether new members will be allowed to join (an open group).

Again, such planning decisions can be taken (a) unilaterally by the facilitator, (b) via negotiation with the group or (c) by the group members only.

Practical Methods of Coping with Stress in the Health Professions: 16

PROBLEM SOLVING

A structured approach to dealing with problems can often help to reduce stress. Adapting the work of Cranwell-Jones (1987), the following stages of problem solving can be identified and worked through:

1. Identify the problem clearly

The more specific you can be about what really is the problem, the better.

2. Collect data of relevance to the problem

You need to list all the relevant facts about all aspects of the problem.

3. Analyse the data you collect

Calm sifting through of all the issues involved will help you to appreciate all sides of the problem. It may help to talk things through with someone else at this stage, too.

4 Generate possible solutions to the problem

Allow yourself to think of ALL possible solutions. Take your time over this stage. The more solutions, both practical and impractical, that you can generate, the better.

5. Evaluate the alternatives and select a solution to the problem

From all the possible solutions, identify the one you want to use.

6. Develop an action plan

Having identified your solution, plan a course of action to achieve it.

7. Implement the action plan

8. Review the outcome

The meaning dimension

This aspect of group facilitation is concerned with what sense group members make of being in the group. As with the previous dimension, at least three options are open here:

1. The facilitator can offer explanations, theories or models to enable group members to make sense of what is happening. Thus a health professional running a support group for bereaved relatives may offer a theoretical model of bereavement to enable those relatives to have a framework for understanding what is happening to them.
2. The facilitator may sometimes offer 'interpretations' of what is going on. At other times, the facilitator will listen to group members' perceptions of what is happening. This may frequently happen in an open discussion group or a case conference.

3. The facilitator offers no explanations or theories but encourages group members to verbalize their own ideas, thoughts and theories. This is the non-directive mode of working with meaning in a group.

The confronting dimension

When people work together, all sorts of conflicts can arise. Sometimes these conflicts are overt and show themselves in arguments and disagreements. Sometimes, a 'hidden agenda' is at work. In this case, conflicts are not made explicit. Instead, they sit just beneath the surface of group life. While they affect it in various ways, they cannot be worked with unless the group addresses them directly. The confronting dimension of facilitation is concerned with ways in which individual members and the group-as-a-whole are challenged. The three ways of working in this dimension are as follows:

1. The facilitator can challenge the group or its members directly by asking questions, making suggestions, or offering interpretations of behaviour in the group. The aim is to encourage the group and its members to confront what is happening at various levels.
2. The health professional can facilitate an atmosphere in which people feel safe enough to challenge each other (and the facilitator). In this process the following 'ground rules' for direct and clear communication can help:

   (a) Say 'I' rather than 'you', 'we' or 'people' when discussing issues in the group.
   (b) Speak directly to other people, rather than about them. Thus 'I am angry with you, David' is better than 'I am angry with people in this group'.
   (c) Take some risks in disclosing what you are thinking or feeling.
3. The facilitator can choose not to confront at all. In this case, two things may happen: (a) no confrontation takes place and the group gets 'stuck', or (b) the group learns to challenge itself, without assistance from the facilitator.

The first option of confrontation, above, is the traditional 'chairperson' mode of facilitation. The health professional who uses this approach stays in control of the group. The negotiated style of confrontation is one that can be used in discussion groups and informal teaching sessions. It can help to encourage autonomy and lessen dependence on the facilitator. The third option is one that can be used in very formal meetings and discussions. If it is used in therapy and self-awareness groups, the chances are that the 'hidden agenda' will not get addressed or that the group members will outgrow the need for the facilitator. It is arguable that *all* groups should aim at becoming independent of the group leader.

The feeling dimension

Therapy groups, self-awareness groups and certain sorts of learning groups tends to generate emotion in participants. The feeling dimension is concerned with how such emotional expression is dealt with. Decisions that can be made in this domain include the following:

1. Will emotional release be *encouraged?* This may be appropriate in a therapy or social skills training group.
2. Is there to be an explicit *contract* with the group about emotional release? Here, the facilitator may suggest at the beginning of the first group meeting that emotional release is 'allowed', thus giving group members permission to express emotions.
3. Does the facilitator feel skilled in handling emotional release? If not, the facilitator may want to develop skills in coping with other people's feelings, especially when these involve the overt expression of tears, anger or fear. Courses in developing such skills are offered at various colleges and universities, including the Human Potential Resource Group at the University of Surrey.

The structuring dimension

Structure is a necessary part of group life. Without it, the group can fall apart. The issues, here, is *how* such structure is developed. Again, at least three options open up in this domain:

1. The facilitator can decide on the total structure of the group. In a social skills group, for example, he or she may introduce a variety of exercises and activities that allow participants to learn how to answer the telephone, introduce themselves at parties or take faulty goods back to a shop. At all times, the facilitator remains in control of the overall structure.
2. The facilitator can encourage group members to organize certain aspects of the life and structure of the group. Thus the ward sister who is running a learning group may invite students to read and discuss seminar papers. In this respect, she is handing over some of the structure to group members.
3. The facilitator can play a minimal role in structuring the life of the group. The extreme example of this is the 'Tavistock' approach to group therapy in which the group starts and finishes at particular times. During the time that the group is running, the facilitator makes no attempt to 'lead' the group. How the people in the group spend the time available is up to them. This is not for the uninitiated!

As a general rule, it is probably better for the new facilitator to start with lots of structure (which is imposed by him or her). As he or she gains confidence in running groups, he or she can gradually hand over some of that structure to group members. This is probably the model that many nursing teachers work to as they develop their careers.

The valuing dimension

This aspect of group facilitation is concerned with creating a supportive and valuing atmosphere in which the group can work. No group will succeed if the atmosphere is one of distrust and suspicion. Nor will continued hostility and disharmony do very much to foster discussion and constructive group work. The issues, here, are the following:

1. Is the facilitator confident enough to allow disagreement, discussion and various points of view?
2. Does the facilitator have sufficient self-awareness to know the effect that he or she is having on the group?
3. Is the facilitator skilled, positive, life asserting and encouraging?

Learning to value other people (and oneself) comes with experience of running groups and developing a range of therapeutic skills such as counselling, social skills and assertiveness. If the facilitator is unable to express warmth, genuineness, and a positive regard for group members, that person is unlikely to be able to create a therapeutic, educational or supportive atmosphere.

Practical Methods of Coping with Stress in the Health Professions: 17

RELAXATION TAPES

Consider buying or preparing a relaxation tape to use when you are very stressed or when you cannot sleep. You can make such a tape by reciting one of the relaxation exercises described in this book into a tape recorder. It has been suggested that the tapes you make yourself are best as you not distracted by an unknown voice and the sound of hearing yourself repeat the stages of relaxation helps to reinforce the process of relaxing.

If you do make your own tape and want to stop during the process of preparing it, use the 'pause' button on the tape recorder. Using the 'stop' button for a short pause will cause an unnerving 'clunk' to be recording which is hardly conducive to relaxation!

SUPERVISION

The process of caring for others can be tiring and emotionally exhausting. Health professionals frequently have to look after the emotional needs of others. When patients have been bereaved or are themselves dying, or when patients are suffering from incurable diseases or are experiencing emotional or psychological upset, all of these factors take their toll on the carer. Health professionals receive little support in the emotional domain, and another approach to coping with stress in caring is via the use of supervision.

Supervision refers to the notion of one health professional acting as a support person for another. The supervisor is one who listens to another, allows freedom of expression and helps in the release of pent-up emotion. As various commentators note (Ellis and Dell, 1986; Holloway, 1984), the role of the supervisor can be extended to include supportive functions such as:

- teaching
- counselling
- evaluation
- befriending.

If the role is extended in these ways, it may be necessary for the person who assumes the role of supervisor to undertake further training in teaching and/or counselling. Sometimes, too, the relationship can be used to enhance personal management skills: self-confidence, decision making and assertiveness (Allan, 1989).

Supervision in practice

How does supervision 'work'? First, a commitment needs to be made between two people: the health professional and the health professional-as-supervisor. Sometimes the person acting as supervisor will be older and more experienced; or will sometimes be a peer, colleague or friend. The relationship need not be one-way. It is quite possible to set up a reciprocal supervisory relationship between two people. In this case, the two people agree to meet regularly for, say, two hours. The first hour of that time is used for one health professional to be supervised by the other. For the second hour, the roles are reversed. This follows the co-counselling format proposed by Heron (1989b). As we have noted, co-counselling is a process in which two people meet for a set period of time. During half of that time, one person acts as 'counsellor' to the other's 'client'. For the other half of the time, the roles are reversed.

Structure

Once agreement that the two health professionals will meet has been achieved, there is need for structure. How will the time be used? For how long will the pair meet and how often? As noted above, in a reciprocal relationship, the two-hour time span is useful. When only one of the pair is acting as supervisor to the

165

other, one hour is probably enough for the meeting. It is recommended that the meetings take place at weekly intervals. It is helpful if the person acting as supervisor uses some basic counselling skills to help to structure the hour, and these have been described in the previous chapter. The supervisor may further structure the supervisory session by using the time available to explore three different domains:

1. How the supervisee is feeling at the moment.
2. What needs to be done next.
3. The supervisee's plans for the next week.

An example may help here. Sarah Jones is a district nurse in a small but busy rural area. She meets her supervisor once a week and the supervisor structures the time according to the above plan. Thus, for the first twenty minutes or so, Sarah talks through her feelings about her work, her patients and her colleagues. During this time, she is free to talk about any aspect of what has happened that week. Needless to say, the supervisory relationship must always be confidential.

During and towards the end of the first twenty-minute period, certain important issues emerge. She reveals that she feels very angry about the way one of her male patients has treated her on recent visits. Sarah feels that the man has been particularly rude and unpleasant. Despite being upset, she has felt, up to this point, that she should try to hide these feelings and to put on a 'professional' front. Gradually, however, she has found that the situation has become more and more stressful.

Once the particular issue has surfaced, the supervisor asks Sarah, 'What has to happen next?'. In the following twenty or so minutes, the pair identify what Sarah has to say or do to resolve her current situation. She realizes that she needs to talk about her feelings on a regular basis. She also begins to appreciate that she needs to become more assertive and be prepared to discuss some of her feelings with the patient in question. In the final twenty-minute period of the hour, Sarah is given help to draw up a definite plan of action. She decides to continue being in supervision on a regular basis. She agrees to talk more to her husband about how she feels about her work. She also plans to discuss with her patient the way that he talks to her on visits. She realizes that this will take tact and will cause her anxiety. Sarah appreciates, though, that the situation will continue unless she takes active steps to do something about it.

This final stage may involve Sarah role-playing what she has to say to her patient and how she will broach the topic of work with her husband. This final stage is important. It is vital that the supervisory period is more than just a 'getting it off your chest' session. The third stage allows for practical action to be planned and taken.

Obviously, this is only *one* approach to structuring supervision and other people may do things differently. The big advantage of structure, however, is that it enables both the supervisor and the person being supervised to feel that they are using their time constructively. It is important that both feel a sense of achievement in what they are doing. Other useful ideas about how to structure the supervisory relationship are offered by Hawkins and Shohet (1989).

Evaluation

It is a good idea for both supervisor and supervisee to look back regularly over the times they have spent together and to identify the way in which the relationship is to develop in the future. This evaluation period can be built into the overall plan of the relationship, right at its start. Thus, both parties agree that they will evaluate the effectiveness of the supervision at monthly intervals.

This raises the question of whether or not notes of the relationship should be kept. If they *are* kept, who should keep them? Again, this issue should be settled before the relationship begins. It is usually better that notes are not taken *during* meetings. Sometimes it is helpful if the health professional keeps a journal of any problems and the ways in which they were resolved. This can either be used as the basis of supervisory sessions or the health professional can keep the journal as a private and confidential record of progress.

Group supervision

So far the discussion has considered only the one-to-one supervisory relationship. A variation on this approach is for a small group

167

of health professionals to agree to meet once a week as a supervision group. The leadership of such a group can 'rotate'. Thus each group meeting is facilitated by a different person each week. Alternatively, the group can agree *not to have a leader*. If this leaderless approach is taken, the following 'ground rules' can help to structure group meetings and avoid their falling into silence or disarray:

- Each person should say 'I' rather than 'you', 'we' or 'people', when relating what has happened to them.
- People should talk *directly* to others. Thus, they should say 'I agree with what you say' rather than 'I agree with what Anne says'.
- Take responsibility for getting what you want from the group. Do not depend on other people to make the group 'work'. Take an active part yourself.

As with one-to-one supervision, the group form of supervision can be structured by using the first twenty-minute period to discuss what has happened during the week, the second twenty-minute period to discuss what has to happen next and the third to draw up plans.

Supervision offers one approach towards helping health professionals to help themselves. If we are to avoid burnout and dissatisfaction, we all need to be able to talk through how we feel about our work, our patients, clients and our colleagues. The structure and sympathetic atmosphere of one-to-one or group supervision can do much to help health professionals to 'offload' and to make practical plans for dealing with future conflict and stress.

SUMMARY

The final chapter of this book has illustrated how a stress reduction workshop can be run. It has also discussed the notion of supervision in the health professions. If we want to take care of others we must first learn to look after ourselves.

Now its over to you. This book has explored a variety of theoretical and practical aspects of stress in the health professions. The question now is: how are *you* coping?

168

Appendix

Values clarification questionnaire

Clarifying our values can help us to deal with the variety of ethical dilemmas that face us in our personal lives and our professional lives as health professionals. Uncertainty over values can add to stress in health professionals as decision making may become difficult.

This questionnaire may be used by a person working alone who wishes to try to identify what he or she holds or does not hold to be important. Alternatively, it can be used in a group or workshop setting as the basis for discussion and values clarification.

Work fairly quickly through the items in the questionnaire, putting a ring around the response that you feel matches your own view most accurately. The possible responses to each item are:

Strongly Agree	SA
Agree	A
Uncertain	U
Disagree	D
Strongly Disagree	SD

1. Clients should be allowed to read their notes.   SA   A   U   D   SD

2. Abortion is always wrong.   SA   A   U   D   SD

3. Religious beliefs should always be respected no matter what the circumstances.   SA   A   U   D   SD

4. Gay people should be allowed to 'marry'.   SA   A   U   D   SD

5. People should be allowed to refuse psychiatric treatment.   SA   A   U   D   SD

6. The individual always knows what is best for her.   SA   A   U   D   SD

7. Wherever possible, children should have two parents.   SA   A   U   D   SD

8. Smokers should be held responsible for
   their own smoking-related diseases.   SA A U D SD

9. I should be able to choose not to work
   with people with AIDS.   SA A U D SD

10. Terminally ill people should have the
    right to end their own lives.   SA A U D SD

11. People are basically good.   SA A U D SD

12. Suicide is always wrong.   SA A U D SD

13. The age of consent should be lowered.   SA A U D SD

14. A nationalized health care system is
    better than a private one.   SA A U D SD

15. All censorship is wrong.   SA A U D SD

16. People should be free to express their
    sexuality according to their preference.   SA A U D SD

17. Certain religious organizations should be
    outlawed.   SA A U D SD

18. The legal system is generally too lenient.   SA A U D SD

19. Psychiatric illness is caused as much by
    social factors as any others.   SA A U D SD

20. Clients should be prepared to pay
    something towards their treatment.   SA A U D SD

21. All children should be offered sex
    education in schools.   SA A U D SD

22. Racial prejudice exists in everyone.   SA A U D SD

23. Political organizations of every
    complexion should be allowed a say on
    television.   SA A U D SD

24. Alcoholics are not 'ill'.   SA A U D SD

25. I agree with most of the policies of the
    present government.   SA A U D SD

26. Parents should be responsible for the
    actions of their children.   SA A U D SD

27. Relatives should always care for sick
    relatives.   SA A U D SD

28. Some religious faiths are 'wrong'.   SA A U D SD

29. Capital punishment should be available
    for certain crimes.   SA A U D SD

30. Contraceptives should be available on
    demand.   SA A U D SD

References

Alberti, R. E. and Emmons, M. L. (1982) *Your Perfect Right: a guide to assertive living*, Impact Publishers, San Louis, California.

Alexander, F. M. (1969) *Resurrection of the Body*, University Books, New York.

Allan, J. (1989) *How to Develop Your Personal Management Skills*, Kogan Page, London.

Atkinson, J. M. (1988) *Coping with Stress at Work: How to Stop Worrying and Start Succeeding*, Thorsons, Wellingborough.

Bailey, R. and Clarke, M. (1989) *Stress and Coping in Nursing*, Chapman and Hall, London.

Bandler, R. and Grinder, J. (1975) *The Structure of Magic 1: A book about language and learning*, Science and Behaviour Books, California.

Bannister, D. and Fransella, F. (1986) *Inquiring Man*, 3rd edn, Croom Helm, London.

Benson, H. (1975) *The Relaxation Response*, Morrow, New York.

Benson, H. (1984) *Beyond the Relaxation Response*, Times Books, New York.

Berne, E. (1972) *What Do You Say After You Say Hello?*, Grove Press, New York

Bernstein, D. A. and Borkovec, T. D. (1973) *Progressive Relaxation Training : a manual for the helping professions*, Research Press, Champaign, Illinois.

Bond, M. (1986) *Stress and Self-Awareness*, Heinemann, London.

Bond, M. and Kilty, J. (1983) *Practical Methods of Coping with Stress*, Human Potential Research Project, University of Surrey, Guildford.

Boud, D. (1981) *Developing Student Autonomy in Learning*, Kogan Page, London.

Brandes, D. (1934) *Becoming a Writer*, Harcourt Brace and Co., London.

Brown, R. (1965) *Social Psychology*, Macmillan, London.

Buber, M. (1958) *I and Thou*, Scribner, New York.

Burnard, P. (1988) The spiritual needs of atheists and agnostics, *The Professional Nurse* **4**, No. 3, 130–2.

Burnard, P. (1989) *Counselling Skills for Health Professionals*, Chapman and Hall, London.

Campbell, A. (1984) *Moderated Love*, SPCK , London.

Canfield, J. and Wells, H. C. (1976) *100 Ways to Enhance Self Concept in the Classroom*, Prentice Hall, Englewood Cliffs, New Jersey.

Cox, M. (1978a) *Structuring the Therapeutic Process*, Pergamon, London.

Cox, T. (1978b) *Stress*, Macmillan, London.

Cranwell-Jones, J. (1987) *Managing Stress*, Gower, Aldershot.

Davis, M., Eshelman, E. R. and McKay, M. (1982) *The Relaxation and Stress Reduction Workbook*, 2nd edn, New Harbinger, Oakland, California.

Egan, G. (1986) *The Skilled Helper*, 3rd edn, Brooks-Cole, Monterey, California.

Ellis, M. V. and Dell, D. M. (1986) Dimensionality of supervisor roles: Supervisor perceptions of supervision, *Journal of Counselling Psychology*, **33**, no. 3, 282–91

Epting, T. R. (1984) *Personal Construct Counselling and Psychotherapy*, Wiley, Chichester.

Ernst, S. and Goodison, L. (1981) *In Our Own Hands: a book of self-help therapy*, The Women's Press, London.

Feldenkrais, M. (1972) *Awareness Through Movement*, Harper and Row, New York.

Firth, J. A. and Shapiro, D. A. (1986) An evaluation of psychotherapy for job-related distress, *Journal of Occupational Psychology*, **59**, 111–19.

Fontana, D. (1989) *Managing Stress*, British Psychological Society and Routledge, London.

Gendlin, E. (1981) *Focusing*, Bantam, New York.

Gunning, R. (1968) *The Technique of Clear Writing*, 2nd edn, McGraw-Hill, London.

Hales-Tooke, J. (1989) Focusing in therapy; focusing in life; self and society, *European Journal of Humanistic Psychology*, **XVII**, no. 6, 113–16.

Hall, C. (1954) *Primer of Freudian Psychology*, Mentor Books, New York.

Hanson, P. (1986) *The Joy of Stress*, Pan, London.

Hargie, O., Saunders, C. and Dickson, D. (1987) *Social Skills in Interpersonal Communication*, 2nd edn, Croom Helm, London.

Hawkins, P. and Shohet, R. (1989) *Supervision in the Helping Professions*, Open University Press, Milton Keynes.

Heron, J. (1970a) *Phenomenology of the Gaze*, Human Potential Research Project, University of Surry, Guildford.

Heron, J. (1970b) *Co-Counselling*, Human Potential Research Project, University of Surrey, Guildford.

Heron, J. (1973) *Experiential Training Techniques*, Human Potential Research Project, University of Surry, Guildford.

Heron, J. (1975) *Six Category Intervention Analysis*, Human Potential Research Project, University of Surry, Guildford.

Heron, J. (1977) *Catharsis in Human Development*, Human Potential Research Project, University of Surry, Guildford.

Heron, J. (1978) *Co-Counselling Teacher's Manual*, Human Potential Research Project, University of Surry, Guildford.

Heron, J. (1981) *Paradigm Papers*, Human Potential Research Project, University of Surrey, Guildford.

Heron, J. (1982) *Education of the Affect*, Human Potential Research Project, University of Surrey, Guildford.

Heron, J. (1986) *Six Category Intervention Analysis*, 2nd edn, Human Potential Research Project, University of Surrey, Guildford.

Heron, J. (1989a) *Six Category Intervention Analysis*, 3rd edn, Human Potential Research Project, University of Surrey, Guildford.

Heron, J. (1989b) *Co-Counselling*, Human Potential Resource Group, University of Surrey, Guildford.

Heron, J. (1989c) *The Facilitators' Handbook*, Kogan Page, London.

Heron, J. and Reason, P. (1982) *A Cooperative Inquiry into Co-Counselling*, Human Potential Research Project, University of Surrey, Guildford.

Hewitt, J. (1977) *Meditation*, Hodder and Stoughton, Sevenoaks, Kent.

Holloway, E. L. (1984) Outcome evaluation in supervision research, *The Counselling Psychologist*, **12**, no. 3, 167–74.

Holmes, T. H. and Rahe, R. H. (1967) The social readjustment rating scale, *Journal of Psychosomatic Research*, **11**, 213–18.

Jackins, H. (1965) *The Human Side of Human Beings*, Rational Island Publishers, Seattle, Washington.

Jackins, H. (1970) *Fundamentals of Co-Counselling Manual*, Rational Island Publishers, Seattle, Washington.

Jick, T. D. (1987) Managing and coping with budget-cut stress in hospitals, in *Stress in Health Professionals*, (eds. R. Payne and J. Firth-Cozens), Wiley, London.

Jones, G. (1987) Stress in psychiatric nursing, in *Stress in Health Professionals*, (eds. R. Payne and J. Firth-Cozens), Wiley, London.

Jourard, S. (1971) *Self-Disclosure: an experimental analysis of the transparent self*, Wiley, New York.

Jung, C. G. (1938) Psychology and religion, in *Collected Works*, vol. 2, Routledge and Kegan Paul, London.

Jung, C. G. (1976) *Modern Man in Search of a Soul*, Routledge and Kegan Paul, London.

Kagan, C. (ed.) (1985) *Interpersonal Skills in Nursing: Research and Applications*, Croom Helm, London.

Kahn, R. L. and Cannell, C. F. (1957) *The Dynamics of Interviewing*, Wiley, New York.

Kelly, G. (1955) *The Psychology of Personal Constructs*, vols 1 and 2, Norton, New York.

Kilty, J. (1983) *Experiential Learning*, Human Potential Research Project, University of Surrey, Guildford.

Kim, M. J., McFarland, G. K. and McLane, A. M. (1987) *Pocket Guide to Nursing Diagnoses*, 2nd ed, C. V. Mosby, St Louis, Missouri.

Kitzinger, S. (1979) *Birth at Home*, Oxford University Press, Oxford.

Knowles, M. S. (1984) *The Adult Learner: a neglected species*, 3rd edn, Gulf, Houston, Texas.

Knowles, M. S. and Associates, (1985) *Andragogy in Action,* Jossey Bass, San Francisco, California.

Laing, R. D. (1959) *The Divided Self*, Penguin, Harmondsworth.

Laing, R. D. (1975) *Knots*, Penguin, Harmondsworth.

Le Shan, L. (1974) *How to Meditate*, Turnstone Press, Wellingborough.

Levine, M. (1982) Methods or madness: on the alienation of the professional, *Journal of Community Psychology*, **10**, 3–14.

Lowen, A. (1967) *Betrayal of the Body*, Macmillan, New York.

Lowen, A. and Lowen, L. (1977) *The Way to Vibrant Health: a manual of bioenergetic exercises*, Harper and Row, New York.

Luft, J. (1969) *Of Human Interaction: The Johari Model*, Mayfield, Palo Alto, California.

Margison, F. R. (1987) Stress in psychiatrists, in *Stress in Health Professionals*, (eds. R. Payne and J. Firth-Cozens), Wiley, London.

REFERENCES

Maslach, C. (1974) Burned out: *Human Behaviour* **5**, 16–22
Maslach, C. (1981) *Burnout: the Cost of Caring*, Prentice Hall, Englewood Cliffs, New Jersey
Maslow, A. (1972) *Motivation and Personality*, Harper and Row, New York.
McCaffery, M. (1979) *Nursing Management of the Patient with Pain*, 2nd edn, Lippincott, Philadelphia, PA.
Meyeroff, M. (1972) *On Caring*, Harper and Row, New York.
Morris, D. (1978) *Manwatching*, Pan, London.
Murgatroyd, S. (1986) *Counselling and Helping*, British Psychological Society and Methuen, London.
Naranjo, C. and Ornstein, R. E. (1971) *On the Psychology of Meditation*, Allen and Unwin, London.
Ornstein, R. E. (1975) *The Psychology of Consciousness*, Penguin, Harmondsworth.
Pearce, J. C. (1982) *The Bond of Power: Meditation and Wholeness*, Routledge and Kegan Paul, London.
Perls, F. (1969a) *Ego, Hunger and Aggression*, Random House, New York.
Perls, F. (1969b) *Gestalt Therapy Verbatim*, Real People Press, Lafayette, California.
Perls, F. S., Hefferline, R. F. and Goodman, P. (1951) *Gestalt Therapy: Excitement and Growth in the Human Personality*, Penguin, Harmondsworth.
Pines, A. M. Aronson, E. and Kafry, D. (1981) *Burnout: from Tedium to Personal Growth*, Free Press, New York.
Reason, P. and Rowan, J. (1981) *Human Inquiry: a sourcebook of new paradigm research*, Wiley, Chichester.
Reich, W. (1949) *Character Analysis*, Simon and Schuster, New York.
Roet, B. (1989) *A Safer Place to Cry*, Macdonald, London.
Rogers, C. R. (1951) *Client Centred Therapy*, Constable, London.
Rogers, C. R. (1967) *On Becoming a Person*, Constable, London.
Rolf, I. (1973) *Structural Integration*, Viking Press, New York.
Rowan, J. (1989) *Subpersonalities*, Routledge, London.
Rushton, A. (1987) Stress amongst social workers, in *Stress in Health Professionals* (eds. R. Payne and J. Firth-Cozens), Wiley, London.
Sartre, J.-P. (1944) *In Camera*, Penguin, Harmondsworth.
Sartre, J.-P. (1956) *Being and Nothingness*, Philosophical Library, New York.
Sartre, J.-P. (1964) *Words*, Penguin, Harmondsworth.
Sartre, J.-P. (1965) *Nausea*, Penguin, Harmondsworth.
Schilling, D. and Poppen, R. (1983) Behavioural relaxation training and assessment, *Journal of Behaviour Therapy and Experimental Psychiatry*, **14**, 99–107.
Schulman, D. (1982) *Intervention in Human Services: a guide to skills and knowledge*, 3rd edn, C. V. Mosby, St Louis, Missouri.
Searle, J. (1983) *Intentionality: an essay in philosophy of mind*, Cambridge University Press, Cambridge.
Selye, H. (1956) *The Stress of Life*, 2nd edn, McGraw-Hill, New York.
Selye, H. (1975) *Stress Without Distress*, Cygnet Books, New York.

Singer, P. (1980) *Marx*, Oxford University Press, Oxford.

Smith, E. and Wilks, N. (1988a) *Meditation*, Optima, London.

Smith, E. and Wilks, N. (1988b) *Meditation*, Macdonald and Co., London.

Spinelli, E. (1989) *The Interpreted World: an Introduction to Phenomenological Psychology*, Sage, London.

Stoll, R. I. (1989) Spirituality and chronic illness, in *Spiritual Dimensions of Nursing Practice*, (ed. V. B. Carson), Saunders, Philadelphia.

Tart, C. (1969) *Altered States of Consciousness*, Wiley, New York.

Terkel, S. (1972) *Working*, Avon Books, New York.

Totton, N. and Edmonston, E. (1988) *Reichian Growth Work: Melting the Blocks to Life and Love*, Prism Press, Bridport.

Vingerhoets, A. J. J. M. and Marcelissen, F. H. G. (1988) Stress research: its present status and issues for future developments, *Social Science and Medicine*, **26**, no.3, 279–91.

Vonnegut, K. (1968) *Mother Night*, Cape, London.

Wallace, A. (1989) An active role for patients in stress management, *The Professional Nurse*, **5**, no. 2, 65–72.

Weil, S. W. and McGill, I. (1989) *Making Sense of Experiential Learning*, Open University Press, Milton Keynes.

Woodcock, M. and Frances, D. (1982) *The Unblocked Manager: a practical guide to self-development*, Gower, Aldershot.

Bibliography

Adams, T. (1989) Dementia and family stress, *Nursing Times*, **85**, no. 38, 27–9.

Addison, C. (1980) Tolerating stress in social work practice: the example of a burns unit, *British Journal of Social Work*, **10**, 341–56.

Alberti, R. (ed.) (1977) *Assertiveness: Innovations, Applications, Issues*, Impact, San Luis, Obispo, California.

Allen, J. (1989) *How to Develop Your Personal Management Skills*, Kogan Page, London.

Anderson, M., Chiriboga, D. A. and Bailey, J. T. (1988) Changes in management stressors on ICU nurses, *Dimensions of Critical Care Nursing*, **7**, no. 2, 111–17.

Argyle, M. (1975) *The Psychology of Interpersonal Behaviour*, Penguin, Harmondsworth.

Argyle, M. (ed.) (1981) *Social Skills and Health*, Methuen, London.

Argyris, C. and Schon, D. (1974) *Theory in Practice: Increasing Professional Effectiveness*, Jossey Bass, San Francisco.

Ascott, M. (1988) Stress in the entertainment business, *Occupational Health*, **40**, no. 4, 520–3.

Ashworth, P. (1987) Technology and machines – bad masters but good servants, *Intensive Care Nursing*, **3**, no. 1, 1–2.

Astbury, C. (1988) *Stress in Theatre Nurses*, Royal College of Nursing, London.

Atwood, A. H. (1979) The mentor in clinical practice, *Nursing Outlook*, **27**, 714–17.

Ausberger, D. (1979) *Anger and Assertiveness in Pastoral Care*, Fortress Press, Philadelphia.

Baer, J. (1976) *How to Be Assertive (Not Aggressive): Women in Life, in Love and on the Job*, Signet, New York.

Bailey, R. (1985) *Coping With Stress in Caring*, Blackwell, Oxford.

Bailey, R. and Clarke, M. (1989) *Stress and Coping in Nursing*, Chapman and Hall, London.

Baker, R. (1984) Stress in welfare work, *National Children's Home Occasional Papers*, No. 5, 1–24.

Bannister, D. and Fransella, F. (1986) *Inquiring Man*, 3rd edn, Croom Helm, London.

Baruth, L. G. (1987) *An Introduction to the Counselling Profession*, Prentice Hall, Englewood Cliffs, New Jersey.

Bates, E. (1982) Doctors and their spouses speak: stress in medical practice, *Sociology of Health and Illness*, **4**, no. 1, 25–39.

Belkin, G. S. (1984) *Introduction to Counselling*, Brown, Dubuque, Iowa.

Bellack, A. S. and Hersen, M. (eds) (1979) *Research and Practice in Social Skills Training*, Plenum Press, New York.

Benner, P. and Wrubel, J. (1989) *The Primacy of Caring: Stress and Coping in Health and Illness*, Addison Wesley, Menlo Park.

Bergman, A. B. (1988) Resident Stress, *Paediatrics*, **82**, no. 2, 260–3.

Bernard, J. M. (1980) Assertiveness in children, *Psychological Reports*, **46**, 935–8.

Bibbings, J. (1987) The stress of working in intensive care: a look at the research, *Nursing*, **3**, no. 15, 567–70.

Bolger, A. W. (ed.) (1982) *Counselling in Britain: a reader*, Batsford Academic, London.

Boud, D., Keogh, R. and Walker, M. (1985) *Reflection: Turning Experience into Learning*, Kogan Page, London.

Bower, S. A. and Bower, G. H. (1976) *Asserting Yourself*, Addison Wesley, Reading, Mass.

Bram, P. J. and Katz, L. F. (1989) A study of burnout in nurses working in hospice and hospital oncology settings, *Oncology Nursing Forum*, **16**, no. 4, 555–60.

Brandes, D. and Phillips, R. (1984) *The Gamester's Handbook*, vol. 2, Hutchinson, London.

Brasweel, M. and Seay, T. (1984) *Approaches to Counselling and Psychotherapy*, Waverly, Prospect Heights.

Brown, A. (1979) *Groupwork*, Heinemann, London.

Brown, D. and Srebalus, D. J. (1988) *An Introduction to the Counselling Process*, Prentice Hall, Philadelphia, PA.

Brown, S. D. and Lent, R. W. (eds) (1984) *Handbook of Counselling Psychology*, Wiley, Chichester.

Buber, M. (1958) *I and Thou*, Scribner, New York.

Buber, M. (1966) *The Knowledge of Man: a philosophy of the interhuman* (ed. M. Freidman; trans. R. G. Smith), Harper and Row, New York.

Bugental, J. F. T. (1980) The far side of despair, *Journal of Humanistic Psychology*, **20**, 49–68.

Bugental, E. K. and Bugental, J. F. T. (1984) Dispiritedness: a new perspective on a familiar state, *Journal of Humanistic Psychology*, **24**, no. 1, 49–67.

Burnard, P. (1987) Spiritual distress and the nursing response: theoretical considerations and counselling skills, *Journal of Advanced Nursing*, **12**, 377–82.

Burnard, P. (1988a) The spiritual needs of atheists and agnostics, *The Professional Nurse*, **4**, no. 3, 130–2.

Burnard, P. (1988) The heart of the counselling relationship, *Senior Nurse*, **8**, no. 12, 17–18.

Burnard, P. (1988b) Stress and relaxation in health visiting, *Health Visitor*, **61**, no. 9, 272.

Burnard, P. (1989) Existentialism as a theoretical basis for counselling in psychiatric nursing, *Archives of Psychiatric Nursing*, **3**, no. 3, 142–7.

Burton, A. (1977) The mentoring dynamic in the therapeutic transformation, *The American Journal of Psychoanalysis*, **37**, 115–22.

Callner, D. and Ross, S. (1978) The assessment and training of assertiveness skills with drug addicts: a preliminary study, *International Journal of the Addictions*, **13**, no. 2, 227–30.

Campbell, A. (1984a) *Paid to Care?*, SPCK, London.

Campbell, A. (1984b) *Moderated Love*, SPCK, London,

Campbell, A. V. (1981) *Rediscovering Pastoral Care*, Darton, Longman and Todd, London.

Carkuff, R. R. (1969) *Helping and Human Relations*, vol. I, *Selection and Training*, Holt, Rinehart and Winston, New York.

Carson, B. V. (1989) *Spiritual Dimensions of Nursing Practice*, Saunders, Philadelphia.

Charles, J. (1983) When carers crash, *Social Work Today*, **15**, no. 12, 18–20.

Cheesebrow, D. J. (1987) Grid analysis for stress management, *Dimensions of Critical Care Nursing*, **6**, no. 5, 314–20.

Chrousos, G. P., Loriaux, D. L. and Gold, P. W. (1988) *Mechanisms of Physical and Emotional Stress*, Plenum Press, New York.

Cianni-Surridge, M. and Horan, J. (1983) On the wisdom of assertive job-seeking behaviour, *Journal of Counselling Psychology*, **30**, 209–14.

Clark, C. (1978) *Assertive Skills for Nurses*, Contemporary Publishing, Wakefield, Mass.

Claxton, G. (1984) *Live and Learn: an introduction to the psychology of growth and change in everyday life*, Harper and Row, London.

Clutterbuck, D. (1985) *Everybody Needs a Mentor: How to Further Talent Within an Organization*, The Institute of Personal Management, London.

Collins, G. C. and Scott, P. (1979) Everyone who makes it has mentor, *Harvard Business Review*, **56**, 89–101.

Cooper, C. L. (1981) *Stress Research*, Wiley, Chichester.

Cooper, C. L. and Marshall, J. (1980) *White Collar and Professional Stress*, Wiley, Chichester.

Cooper, C. L. and Payne, R. (eds) (1978) *Stress at Work*, Wiley, Chichester.

Cooper, C. L. and Payne, R. (1980) *Current Concerns in Occupational Stress*, Wiley, Chichester.

Corey, F. (1983) *I Never Knew I Had A Choice*, 2nd edn, Brooks-Cole, California.

Cormier, L. S. (1987) *The Professional Counsellor: a process guide to helping*, Prentice Hall, Englewood Cliffs, New Jersey.

Corsini, R. (1984) *Current Psychotherapies*, 3rd edn, Peacock, Itasca, Illinois.

Cunningham, P. M. (1983) Helping students extract meaning from experience, in *Helping Adults Learn How to Learn: New Directions for Continuing Education* (ed. R. M. Smith), no. 19, Jossey Bass, San Francisco.

Curtis, L., Sturm, G., Billing, D. R. and Anderson, J. D. (1989) At the breaking point; when should an overworked nurse bail out?, *Journal of Christian Nursing*, **6**, no. 1, 4–9.

Daleo, R. E. (1986) Taking care of the caregivers: five strategies for stamina, *American Journal of Hospice Care*, **3**, no. 5, 33–8.

Darling, L. A. W. (1984) What do nurses want in a mentor? *The Journal of Nursing Administration*, October, 42–4.

Darling, L. W. (1986) What to do about toxic mentors, *Nurse Educator*, **11**, no. 2, 29–30.

Dawley, H. and Wenrich, W. (1976) *Achieving Assertive Behaviour: a guide to assertive training*, Brooks-Cole, Monterey, California.

Deckard, G. J. (1989) Impact of role stress on physical therapists' emotional and physical well-being, *Physical Therapist*, **69**, no. 9, 713–18.

Dewe, P. J. (1989) Stressor frequency, tension, tiredness and coping: some measurement issues and a comparison across nursing groups, *Journal of Advanced Nursing*, **14**, no. 4, 308–20.

Dickson, A. (1985) *A Woman in Your Own Right: Assertiveness and You*, Quartet Books, London.

Dilts, P. V. Jr, and Dilts, S. L. (1987) Stress in residency: proposals for solution, *American Journal of Obstetrics and Gynaecology*, **157**, no. 5, 1093–6.

Distance Learning Centre (1986) *Stress in Nursing: an open learning study pack*, Distance Learning Centre, South Bank Polytechnic, London.

Dixon, D. N. and Glover, J. A. (1984) *Counselling: a problem solving approach*, Wiley, Chichester.

Dobson, C. B. (1982) *Stress: The Hidden Anxiety*, MTP Press, Lancaster.

Dolan, N. (1987) The relationship between burnout and job satisfaction in nurses, *Journal of Advanced Nursing*, **12**, no. 1, 3–12.

Doswell, W. M. (1989) Physiological responses to stress, *Annual Review of Nursing Research*, **7**, 51–69.

Douglas, T. (1979) *Groupwork Practice*, Tavistock, London.

Downe, S. (1989) Prophets without honour – the burn-out of midwifery visionaries, *Midwives Chronicle*, **102**, no. 1214, 93–4.

Duncan, S. and Fiske, D. W. (1977) *Face-to-Face Interaction: Research, Methods and Theory*, Lawrence Erlbaum Associates, Hillsdale, New Jersey.

Edelwich, J. Brondsky, A. (1980) *Burnout: Stages of Disillusionment in the Helping Professions*, Human Sciences Press, New York.

Eden, D. (1982) Critical job events, acute stress and strain, *Organizational Behaviour and Human Performance*, **30**, 312–29.

Egan, G. (1986a) *Exercises in Helping Skills*, 3rd edn, Brooks-Cole, Monterey, California.

Egan, G. (1986b) *The Skilled Helper*, 3rd edn, Brooks-Cole, Monterey, California.

Ellis, A. (1962) *Reason and Emotion in Psychotherapy*, Lyle, Stuart, New Jersey.

Ellis, R. and Whittington, D. (1981) *A Guide to Social Skill Training*, Croom Helm, London.

Ellis, R. and Whittington, D. (eds) (1983) *New Directions in Social Skills Training*, Croom Helm, London.

Epting, F. (1984) *Personal Construct Counselling and Psychotherapy*, Wiley, Chichester.

Everly, G. S. and Rosenfeld, R. (1981) *The Nature and Treatment of the Stress Response: a practical guide for clinicians*, Plenum Press, New York.

Fabry, J. (1968) *The Pursuit of Meaning*, Beacon Press, Boston, Mass.

Fagan, M. M. and Walter, G. (1982) Mentoring among teachers, *Journal of Educational Research*, **76**, no. 2, 113–18.

Farber, B. A. (ed.) (1983) *Stress and Burnout in the Human Services*, Pergamon Press, London.

179

Fay, A. (1978) *Making Things Better by Making Them Worse*, Hawthorne, New York.

Feldenkrais, M. (1972) *Awareness Through Movement*, Harper and Row, New York.

Ferruci, P. (1982) *What We May Be*, Turnstone Press, Wellingborough.

Fineman, S. (1985) *Social Work Stress and Intervention*, Gower, London.

Firth, J. (1985) Personal meanings of occupational stress: cases from the clinic, *Journal of Occupational Psychology*, **58**, 139–48.

Firth, J. A. (1986) Levels and sources of stress in medical students, *British Medical Journal*, **292**, 1177–80.

Firth, H., McKeown, P., McIntee, J. and Britton, P. (1987) Burnout, personality and support in long-stay nursing, *Nursing Times*, **83**, no. 32, 55–7.

Fisher, S. (1986) *Stress and Strategy*, Lawrence Erlbaum Associates, London.

Fisher, S. and Reason, J. (1988) *Handbook of Life Stress: Cognition and Health*, Wiley, Chichester.

Foggo-Pays, E. (1983) *An Introductory Guide to Counselling*, Ravenswood, Beckenham.

Fordham, F. (1966) *An Introduction to Jung's Psychology*, Penguin, Harmondsworth.

France, R. and Robson, M. (1986) *Behaviour Therapy in Primary Care*.

Francis, D. and Young, D. (1979) *Improving Work Groups: a practical manual for team building*, University Associates, San Diego, California.

Frankl, V. E. (1959) *Man's Search for Meaning*, Beacon Press, New York.

Frankl, V. E. (1960) Paradoxical intention: a logotherapeutic technique, *American Journal of Psychotherapy*, **14**, 520–35.

Frankl, V. E. (1969) *The Will to Meaning*, World Publishing Co., New York.

Frankl, V. E. (1975a) Paradoxical intention and dereflection: a logotherapeutic technique, *Psychotherapy: Theory, Research and Practice*, **12**, no. 3, 226–37.

Frankl, V. E. (1975b) *The Unconscious God*, Simon and Schuster, New York.

Frankl, V. E. (1978) *The Unheard Cry for Meaning*, Simon and Schuster, New York.

French, P. (1983) *Social Skills for Nursing Practice*, Croom Helm, London.

Freudenberger, H. and Richelson, G. (1974) *Burnout: How to Beat the High Cost of Success*, Bantam Books, New York.

Fromm, E. (1941) *Escape from Freedom*, Avon, New York.

Geller, L. (1985) Another look at self-actualization, *Journal of Humanistic Psychology*, **24**, no. 2, 93–106.

Gendlin, E. T. and Beebe, J. (1968) An experiential approach to group therapy, *Journal of Research and Developments in Education*, **1**, 19–29.

George, P. and Kummerow, J. (1981) Mentoring for career women, *Training*, **18**, no. 2, 44–9.

Gibson, R. L. and Mitchell, M. H. (1986) *Introduction to Counselling and Guidance*, Collier Macmillan, London.

Gier, M. D., Levick, M. D. and Blazina, P. J. (1988) Stress reduction with heart transplant patients and their families: a multidisciplinary approach, *Journal of Heart Transplantation*, **7**, no. 5, 342–7.

Gilleard, C.J. (1987) Influence of emotional distress among supporters on the outcome of psychogeriatric day care, *British Journal of Psychiatry*, **150**, 219–23.

Goffman, I. (1971) *The Presentation of Self in Everday Life*, Penguin, Harmondsworth.

Goldberg, L. and Beznitz, S. (1982) *Handbook of Stress: Theoretical and Clinical Aspects*, Macmillan, New York.

Gordon, S. and Waldo, M. (1984) The effects of assertive training on couples' relationships, *American Journal of Family Therapy*, **12**, 73–7.

Gormally, J. (1982) Evaluation of assertiveness: effects of gender, Rate of involvement and level of assertiveness, *Behaviour Therapy*, **13**, 219–25.

Graham, N. M. (1988) Psychological stress as a public health problem: how much do we know?, *Community Health Studies*, **12**, no. 2, 151–60.

Haggerty, L. A. (1987) An analysis of senior nursing students' immediate responses to distressed patients, *Journal of Advanced Nursing*, **12**, no. 4, 451–61.

Halmos, P. (1965) *The Faith of the Counsellors*, Constable, London.

Hamilton, M. S. (1981) Mentorhood: a key to nursing leadership, *Nursing Leadership*, **4**, no. 1, 4–13.

Hanks, L, Belliston, L. and Edwards, D. (1977) *Design Yourself*, Kaufman, Los Altos, California.

Hargie, O., Saunders, C. and Dickson, D. (1981) *Social Skills in Interpersonal Communication*, 2nd edn, Croom Helm, London.

Harris, T. (1969) *I'm O.K., You're O.K.*, Harper and Row, London.

Health Education Authority (1988) *Stress in the Public Sector: Nurses, Police, Social Workers and Teachers*, High Stress Occupation Working Party, Health Education Authority.

Heins, M., Fahey, S. N. and Leiden, L. I. (1984) Perceived stress in medical, law and graduate students, *Journal of Medical Education*, **59**, 169–79.

Hemmons, J. (1986) Stress in OH nursing?, *Occupational Health*, **38**, no. 10, 328–30.

Herinck, R. (ed.) (1980) *The Psychotherapy Handbook*, New American Library, New York.

Heron, J. (1977a) *Catharsis in Human Development*, Human Potential Research Project, University of Surrey, Guildford.

Heron, J. (1977b) *Behaviour Analysis in Education and Training*, Human Potential Research Project, University of Surrey, Guildford.

Hingley, P. and Cooper, C. L. (1986) *Stress and the Nurse Manager*, Wiley, Chichester.

Holt, R. (1982) An alternative to mentorship, *Adult Education*, **55**, no. 2, 152–6.

Hughes, J. (1987) *Cancer and Emotion*, Wiley, Chichester.

Hull, D. and Schroeder, H. (1979) Some interpersonal effects of assertion, non-assertion and aggression, *Behaviour Therapy*, **10**, 20–9.

Hurding, R. F. (1985) *Roots and Shoots: a guide to counselling and psychotherapy*, Hodder and Stoughton, London.

Hutchins, D. E. (1987) *Helping Relationships and Strategies*, Brooks-Cole, Monterey, California.

Ivey, A. E, (1987) *Counselling and Psychotherapy: Skills, Theories and Practice*, Prentice Hall International, London.

Jacobson, D. (1989) Context and the sociological study of stress: an invited response to Pearlin, *Journal of Health and Social Behaviour*, **30**, no. 3, 257–60.

Jacobson, S. F. (1983) Stresses and coping strategies of neonatal intensive care unit nurses, *Research in Nursing and Health Practitioner*, **226**, 1580–2.

James, M. and Jongeward, D. (1971) *Born to Win: transactional analysis with Gestalt experiments*, Addison-Wesley, Reading, Mass.

Jenkins, E. (1987) *Facilitating Self-Awareness: a learning package combining group work with computer assisted learning*, Open Software Library, Wigan.

Jenkins, J. F. and Ostchega, Y. (1986) Evaluation of burnout in oncology nurses, *Cancer Nursing*, **9**, no. 3, 108–16.

Johnson, D. W. and Johnson, F. P. (1982) *Joining Together*, 2nd edn, Prentice Hall, Englewood Cliffs, New Jersey.

Jones, G. (1988) High-tech stress: identification and prevention, *Occupational Health*, **40**, no. 9, 648–9.

Jones, J. G., Janman, K., Payne, R. L. and Rick, J. T. (1987) Some determinants of stress in psychiatric nurses, *International Journal of Nursing Studies*, **24**, no. 2, 129–44.

Jourard, S. (1964) *The Transparent Self*, Van Nostrand, Princeton, New Jersey.

Jourard, S. (1971) *Self-Disclosure: an experimental analysis of the transparent self*, Wiley, New York.

Kampel, W. and Kampel, M. (1988) Dental stress. The way it was/The way it is, *Alpha-Omegan*, **81**, no. 1, 18–19.

Kavanagh, K. H. (1989) Nurses' networks: obstacles and challenge, *Archives of Psychiatric Nursing*, **3**, no. 4, 226–33.

Keller, K. L. and Koenig, W. J. (1989) Sources of stress and satisfaction in emergency practice, *Journal of Emergency Medicine*, **7**, no. 3, 293–9.

Kelly, C. (1979) *Assertion Training: a facilitator's guide*, University Associates, La Jolla, California.

Kennedy, E. (1979) *On Becoming a Counsellor*, Gill and Macmillan, London.

Koberg, D. and Bagnal, J. (1981) *The Rivised All New Universal Traveller: a soft-systems guide to creativity, problem-solving and the process of reaching goals*, Kaufmann, Los Altos, California.

Kopp, S. (1974) *If You Meet the Buddha on the Road, Kill him!: a modern pilgrimage through myth, legend and psychotherapy*, Sheldon Press, London.

Kottler, J. A. and Brown, R. W. (1985) *Introduction to Therapeutic Counselling*, Brooks-Cole, Monterey, California.

L'Abate, L. and Milan, M. (eds) (1985) *Handbook of Social Skills Training and Research*, Wiley, New York.

Lachman, V. D. (1983) *Stress Management: a manual for nurses*, Grune and Stratton, Orlando, Florida.

Lang, A. J. and Jakubowski, P. (1978) *The Assertive Option*, Research Press, Champagne.

Larson, D. G. (1986) Developing effective hospice staff support groups: pilot test of an innovative training programs, *Hospice Journal*, **2**, no. 2, 41–55.

Lazarus, R. S. and Folkman, S. (1984) *Stress, Appraising and Coping*, Springer, New York.

Leady, N. K. (1989) A physiological analysis of stress and chronic illness, *Journal of Advanced Nursing*, **14**, no. 10, 868–76.

Leech, K. (1986) *Spirituality and Pastoral Care*, Sheldon Press, London.

Lennon, M. C. (1989) The structural contexts of stress: an invited response to Pearlin, *Journal of Health and Social Behaviour*, **30**, no. 3, 261–8.

Lewis, H. and Streitfield, H. (1971) *Growth Games*, Bantam Books, New York.

Lewis, M. (1987) *Writing to Win*, McGraw-Hill, London.

Liberman, R. P., King, L. W., DeRisi, W. J. and McCann, M. (1976) *Personal Effectiveness*, Research Press, Champagne.

Luft, J. (1984) *Group Processes: an introduction to group dynamics*, 2nd edn, Mayfield, San Francisco.

Lyon, B. L. and Werner, J. S. (1987) Research on nursing practice: stress, *Annual Review of Nursing Research*, **5**, 3–22.

Madders, J. (1980) *Stress and Relaxation*, Martin Dunitz, London.

Magrath, A., Reid, N. and Boore, J. (1989) Occupation stress in nursing, *International Journal of Nursing Studies*, **26**, no. 4, 343–58.

Marshall, E. K. and Kurtz, P. D. (eds) (1982) *Interpersonal Helping Skills: a guide to training methods, programs and resources*, Jossey Bass, San Francisco, California.

Matthews, D. A., Classen, D. C., Willms, J. L. and Cotton, J. P. (1988) A program to help interns cope with stresses in an internal medicine residency, *Journal of Medical Education*, **63**, no. 7, 539–47.

May, K. M. *et al.* (1982) Mentorship for scholarliness: opportunities and dilemmas, *Nursing Outlook*, **30**, 22–8.

McCue, J. D. (1986) Doctors and stress: is there really a problem?, *Hospital Practice*, 30 March, 7–16.

McGuire, J. and Priestley, P. (1981) *Life After School: a social skills curriculum*, Pergamon, Oxford.

McIntee, J. and Firth, H. (1984) How to beat the burnout, *Health and Social Services Journal*, 9 February, 166–8.

Meichenbaum, D. (1979) *Cognitive Behaviour Modification: an integrative approach*, Plenum Press, New York.

Meichenbaum, D. (1983) *Coping With Stress*, Century Publishing, London.

Meichenbaum, D. and Jaremko, M. E. (1983) *Stress Reduction and Prevention*, Plenum Press, New York.

Merriam, S. (1984) Mentors and proteges: a critical review of the literature, *Adult Education Quarterly*, **33**, no. 3, 161–73.

Middleton, J. F. (1989) Modifying the behaviour of doctors and their receptionists in recurrent stressful activity, *Journal of the Royal College of General Practitioners*, **39**, no. 319, 62–4.

Milne, D., Burdett, C. and Beckett, J. (1986) Assessing and reducing the stress and strain of psychiatric nursing, *Nursing Times*, **82**, no. 19, 59–62.

Moore, D. (1977) *Assertive Behaviour Training: an annotated bibliography*, Impact, San Luis, Obispo, California.

Moreno, J. L. (1959) *Psychodrama*, vol. II, Beacon House Press, Beacon, New York.

Moreno, J. L. (1969) *Psychodrama*, vol. III, Beacon House Press, Beacon, New York.

Moreno, J. L. (1977) *Psychodrama*, vol. I, 4th edn, Beacon House Press, Beacon, New York.

Morsund, J. (1985) *The Process of Counselling and Therapy*, Prentice Hall, Englewood Cliffs, New Jersey.

Mouton, J. S. and Blake, R. R. (1984) *Synergogy: a new strategy for education, training and development*, Jossey Bass, San Francisco, California.

Muller, P. A. (1987) Avoiding burnout through prevention, *Journal of Post Anaesthetic Nursing*, **2**, no. 1, 53–8.

Munro, A., Manthei, B. and Small, J. (1988) *Counselling: The Skills of Problem-Solving*, Routledge, London.

Murgatroyd, S. and Woolfe, R. (1982) *Coping with Crisis – Understanding and Helping Persons in Need*, Harper and Row, London.

Murphy, J. M., Nadelson, C. C. and Notman, M. T. (1984) Factors influencing first-year medical students' perceptions of stress, *Journal of Human Stress*, **10**, 165–73.

Murphy, L. R. (1984) Occupational stress management: a review and appraisal, *Journal of Occupational Psychology*, **57**, 1–15.

Murphy, S. A. (1986) Perceptions of stress, coping and recovery one and three years after a natural disaster, *Issues in Mental Health Nursing*, **8**, no. 1, 63–77.

Myerscough, P. R. (1989) *Talking With Patients: a basic clinical skill*, Oxford Medical Publications, Oxford.

Nadler, L. (ed.) (1984) *The Handbook of Human Resource Development*, Wiley, New York.

Nash, E. S. (1989) Occupational stress and the oncology nurse, *Nursing*, **4**, no. 8, 37–8.

Nelson-Jones, R. (1981) *The Theory and Practice of Counselling Psychology*, Holt, Rinehart and Winston, London.

Nelson-Jones, R. (1983) *Practical Counselling Skills: a psychological skills approach for the helping professions and for voluntary counsellors*, Holt, Rinehart and Winston, London.

Nelson-Jones, R. (1984) *Personal Responsibility: Counselling and Therapy, an integrative approach*, Harper and Row, London.

Nelson-Jones, R. (1988) *Practical Counselling and Helping Skills: helping clients to help themselves*, Cassell, London.

Notman, M. T., Salt, P, and Nadelson, C. C. (1984) Stress and adaptation in medical students: who is most vulnerable?, *Comprehensive Psychiatry*, **25**, 355–66.

Nutall, P. (1982) Take me to your mentor, *Nursing Times*, **78**, no. 20, 826.

O'Dowd, T. C. (1987) To burn out or to rust out in general practice, *Journal of the Royal College of General Practice*, **37**, no. 300, 290–1.

Ohlsen, A. M., Horne, A. M. and Lawe, C. F. (1988) *Group Counselling*, Holt, Rinehart and Winston, New York.

Onady, A. A., Rodenhauser, P. and Market, R. J. (1988) Effects of stress and social phobia on medical students' specialty choices, *Journal of Medical Education*, **63**, no. 3, 162–70.

Open University Coping With Crisis Group (1987) *Running Workshops: a guide for trainers in the helping professions*, Croom Helm, London.

Osborn, S. M. and Harris, G. G. (1975) *Assertive Training for Women*, Charles C. Thomas, Springfield, Illinois.

Palmer, M. E. and Deck, E. S. (1982) Assertiveness education: one method for teaching staff and patients, *Nurse Educator*, Winter, 36–9.

Payne, R. and Firth-Cozens, J. (eds) (1987) *Stress in Health Professionals*, Wiley, Chichester.

Pearlin, L. I. (1989) The sociological study of stress, *Journal of Health and Social Behaviour*, **30**, no. 3, 241–56.

Phelps, S. and Austin, N. (1975) *The Assertive Woman*, Impact, San Luis, Obispo, California.

Phillip-Jones, L. (1982) *Mentors and Proteges*, Arbour House, New York.

Phillip-Jones, L. (1983) Establishing a formalized mentoring programme, *Training and Development Journal*, February, 38–42.

Pollack, K. (1988) On the nature of social stress: production of a modern mythology, *Social Science and Medicine*, **26**, no. 3, 381–92.

Pope, B. (1986) *Social Skills Training for Psychiatric Nurses*, Harper and Row, London.

Priestley, P., McQuire, J., Flegg, D., Hemsley, V. and Welham, D. (1978) *Social Skills and Personal Problem Solving*, Tavistock, London.

Procter, B. (1978) *Counselling Shop: an introduction to the theories and techniques of ten approaches to counselling*, Deutsch, London.

Rawlings, M. E. and Rawlings, L. (1983) Mentoring and networking for helping professionals, *Personnel and Guidance Journal*, **62**, 2, 116–18.

Reddy, M. (1987) *The Manager's Guide to Counselling at Work*, Methuen, London.

Roche, G. R. (1979) Much ado about mentors, *Harvard Business Review*, **56**, 14–28.

Rogers, C. R. (1951) *Client-Centred Therapy*, Constable, London.

Rogers, C. R. (1967) *On Becoming a Person*, Constable, London.

Rogers, C. R. (1983) *Freedom to Learn for the Eighties*, Merrill, Columbus.

Rogers, C. R. (1985) Toward a more human science of the person, *Journal of Humanistic Psychology*, **25**, no. 4, 7–24.

Rogers, C. R. and Stevens, B. (1967) *Person to Person: The Problem of Being Human*, Real People Press, Lafayette, California.

Rogers, J. C. (1982) Sponsorship – developing leaders for occupational therapy, *American Journal of Occupational Therapy*, **36**, 309–13.

Rogers, J. C. and Dodson, S. C. (1988) Burnout in occupational therapists, *Americal Journal of Occupational Therapy*, **42**, no. 12, 787–92.

Rowan, J. (1986) Holistic listening, *Journal of Humanistic Psychology*, **26**, no. 1, 83–102.

Scharer, K. (1988) Care for the care-giver, *Journal of the Association of Paediatric Oncology Nurses*, **5**, nos 1–2, 24.

Schmidt, J. A. and Wolfe, J. S. (1980) The mentor partnership: discovery of professionalism, *NASPA Journal*, **17**, 45–51.

Schon, D. A. (1983) *The Reflective Practitioner: How Professionals Think in Action*, Basic Books, New York.

Schorr, T. M. (1978) The lost art of mentoring, *American Journal of Nursing*, **78**, 1873.

Schulman, D. (1982) *Intervention in Human Services: a guide to skills and knowledge*, 3rd edn, C. V. Mosby, St Louis, Missouri.

Shafer, P. (1978) *Humanistic Psychology*, Prentice Hall, Englewood Cliffs, New Jersey.

Shamian, J. and Inhaber, R. (1985) The concept and practice of preceptorship in contemporary nursing: a review of pertinent literature, *The International Journal of Nursing Studies*, **22**, no. 2, 79–88.

Shapiro, E. C., Haseltime, F. and Rowe, M. (1978) Moving up: role models, mentors and the patron system, *Sloan Management Review*, **19**, 51–8.

Shaw, M. E. (1981) *Group Dynamics: the psychology of small group behaviour*, McGraw-Hill, New York.

Shostak, A. B. (1980) *Blue-Collar Stress*, Addison-Wesley, Reading Mass.

Shropshire, C. O. (1981) Group experiential learning in adult education, *The Journal of Continuing Education in Nursing*, **12**, no. 6, 5–9.

Simon, S. B., Howe, L. W. and Kirschenbaum, H. (1978) *Values Clarification*, rev. edn, A. and W. Visual Library, New York.

Smith, T. (1984) Stress in the prison service, *Prison Service Journal*, October, 10–11.

Speizer, J. J. (1981) Role models, mentors and sponsors: the elusive concept, *Signs*, **6**, 692–712.

Stevens, J. O. (1971) *Awareness: Exploring, Experimenting, Experiencing*, Real People Press, Moab, Utah.

Taubman, B. (1976) *How to Become an Assertive Woman*, Simon and Schuster, New York.

Taylor, S. (1986) Mentors: who are they and what are they doing?, *Thrust for Educational Leadership*, **15**, no. 7, 39–41.

Taylor, E. (1988) Anger intervention, *American Journal of Occupational Therapy*, **42**, no. 3, 147–55.

Thompson, J. (1989) Stress sense, *Nursing Times*, **85**, no. 21, 20.

Tough, A. M. (1982) *Intentional Changes: a fresh approach to helping people change*, Cambridge Books, New York.

Trower, P., Bryant, B. M. and Argyle, M. (eds) (1978) *Social Skills and Mental Health*, Methuen, London.

Trower, P., O'Mahony, J. M. and Dryden, W. (1982) Cognitive aspects of social failure: some implications for social skills training, *British Journal of Guidance and Couselling*, **10**, 176–84.

Truax, C. B. and Carkuff, R. P. (1967) *Towards Effective Counselling and Psychotherapy*, Aldine, Chicago.

Vredenburg, D. J. and Trinkause, R. J. (1983) An analysis of role stress among hospital nurses, *Journal of Vocational Behaviour*, **22**, 82–95.

Wallace, W. A. (1986) *Theories of Counselling and Psychotherapy: a basic issues approach*, Allyn and Bacon, Boston.

Wallis, R. (1984) *Elementary Forms of the New Religious Life*, Routledge and Kegan Paul, London.

Watkins, J. (1978) *The Therapeutic Self*, Human Science Press, New York.

Weatley, D. (1981) *Stress and the Heart: interactions of the cardiovascular system, behaviour states and psychotropic drugs*, Raven Press, New York.

Wheeler, D. D. and Janis, I. L. (1980) *A Practical Guide for Making Decisions*, Free Press, New York.

Whitaker, D. S. (1985) *Using Groups to Help People*, Tavistock/Routledge, London.

Wilkinson, J., and Canter, S. (1982) *Social Skills Training Manual: assessment, programme design and management of training*, Wiley, Chichester.

Winn, M. F. (1988) Imagery and the school nurse, *Journal of School Health*, **58**, no. 3, 112–14.

Wlodkowski, R. J. (1985) *Enhancing Adult Motivation to Learn*, Jossey Bass, San Francisco, California.

Zander, A. (1982) *Making Groups Effective*, Jossey Bass, San Francisco, California.

Zastrow, C. (1984) Understanding and preventing burnout, *British Journal of Social Work*, **14**, 141–55.

Index

Acceptance 24
Accomplishment, reduced
personal 9
Adams, T. 176
Addison, C. 176
Alberti, R. E. and Emmons, M.
L. 104, 171
Alexander, F. M. 51, 129, 171
Alexander technique 51, 129
Alienation 34
Allan, J. 165, 171
Allport, G. 37
Altshuler, J. L. 176
Anderson, M., Chiriboga, D. A.
and Bailey, J. T. 176
Approaches to stress 3
Argyle, M. 176
Argyris, C. and Schon, D. 176
Ascott, M. 176
Ashworth, P. 176
Aspects of self 36
Assertion 79, 98–100
Assessing life stress 115
Assessing your stress levels 111
Astbury, C. 176
Atkinson, J. M. 171
Attending 123
Atwood, A. H. 176
Ausberger, D. 176
Authenticity 33
Awareness of problems 10

Baer, J. 176
Bailey, R. and Clarke, M. 3, 171,
176
Baker, R. 176
Bandler, R. and Grinder, J. 44,
105, 171
Bannister, D. and Fransella, F.
37, 171
Baruth, L. G. 176

Bates, E. 176
Behavioural relaxation
training 121
Belkin, G. S. 176
Bellack, A. S. and Hersen,
M. 176
Benner, P. and Wrubel, J. 176
Benson, H. 84, 91, 94, 171
Bergman, A. B. 176
Bernard, J. M. 177
Berne, E. 89, 90, 171
Bernstein, D. A. and Borkovec,
T. D. 83, 171
Bibbings, J. 177
Bioenergetics 22
Blind area, the 55
Blocked emotions 21, 146
Body language 128
Body, experience of the 49
Bodywork 51, 55
Bolger, A. W. 177
Bond, M. 43, 47, 54, 141, 152,
155, 171
Bond, M. and Kilty, J. 47, 117,
155, 171
Bottled up emotions 16, 21, 27,
30
Boud, D., Keogh, R. and Walker,
M. 177
Boud, D. 145, 171
Bower, S. A. and Bower,
G. H., 177
Brainstorming 111
Bram, P. J. and Katz, L. F. 177
Brandes, D. 92, 171
Brandes, D. and Phillips, R. 177
Brasweel, M. and Seay, T. 177
Breathing techniques 76–80
Breathing square, the 78
Breathing exercise 23
Brown, A. 177

Brown, S. D. and Lent, R. W. 177
Brown, D. and Srebalus, D. J. 177
Brown, R. 43, 171
Buber, M. 34, 171
Buddhist mantra 95
Bugental, J. F. T. 177
Bugental, E. K. and Bugental, J. F. T. 177
Burnard, P. 53, 54, 88, 171
Burnout 7, 8, 51

Callner, D. and Ross, S. 177
Calming techniques 92
Campbell, A. 171, 177
Canfield, J. and Wells, H. C. 75, 171
Carkuff, R. R. 178
Carson, B. V. 178
Cartesian dualism 45
Causes of stress 117
Character analysis 64
Charles, J. 178
Checking for understanding 134, 143
Cheesebrow, D. J. 178
Children's wards 145
Christian mantra 94
Chrousos, G. P., Loriaux, D. L. and Gold, P. W. 178
Church workers 90
Cianni-Surridge, M. and Horan, J. 178
Clark, C. 178
Clarke, M. 3
Claxton, G. 178
Client-centred counselling 133
Clinical depression 90
Closed questions 135
Clutterbuck, D. 178
Co-counselling 47, 54, 122, 144–7
Cognitive clarity 11
Collins, G. C. and Scott, P. 178
Confrontation 109

Confronting questions 138
Conscious use of the self 45
Contradiction 29
Control 25
Cooper, C. L. and Payne, R. 178
Coping with stress 12, 117
Coping skills 12
Corey, F. 178
Cormier, L. S. 178
Corsini, R. 178
Counselling 122, 123, 127, 132, 155
Cox, M. 171
Cox, T. 2, 171
Cranwell-Jones, J. 171
Creativity 48
Criteria for personhood 37
Culture 105
Cultural differences 43
Cunningham, P. M. 178
Curtis, L., Sturm, G., Billing, D. R. and Anderson, J. D. 178

Daleo, R. E.
Darker aspects of self 38
Darling, L. A. W. 178
Davis, M., Eshelman, E. R. and McKay, M. 79, 171
Dawley, H. and Wenrich, W. 179
Decision-making, difficult in 22
Deckard, G. J. 179
Depersonalization 9
Depression, clinical 90
Descartes, R. 45
Determinism 35
Dewe, P. J. 179
Dickson, A. 179
Dilts, P. V. Jr, and Dilts, S. L. 179
Dimensions of facilitation 157
Dispiritedness 87
Displacement 24
Distance Learning Centre 179
Dixon, D. N. and Glover, J. A. 179

Dobson, C. B. 179
Dolan, N. 179
Doswell, W. M. 179
Douglas, T. 179
Downe, S. 179
Duncan, S. and Fiske, D. W. 179

Early memories 28
Eastern philosophy 64
Echoing 140
Edelwich, J. and Brondsky,
    A. 179
Eden, D. 179
Egan, G. 130, 171
Ego boundaries 58, 62
Ellis, A. 179
Ellis, R. and Whittington, D. 179
Ellis, M. V. and Dell,
    D. M. 164–5, 172
Emotion
    bottled up 16, 21, 30
    positive use of 26
Emotional
    aspect of the person 46
    exhaustion 9
    release 31
Emotions, the nature of 15
Empathy building 134, 142
Environmental factors in
    stress 113
Epting, T. R. 172
Ernst, S. and Goodison, L. 75,
    127, 172
Evaluation 167
Everly G. S. and Rosenfeld,
    R. 179
Existential philosophy 32
Experience of the body 49
Eye contact 43, 104

Fabry, J. 179
Facial expression 105
Facilitating support groups 157
Fagan, M. M. and Walter, G. 179
Fantasy 124–5
Farber, B. A. 180

Faulty beliefs 23
Faulty self-image 22
Fay, A. 180
Feeling 21
Feeling dimension, the 46
Feelings, stress and 15–30
Feldenkrais, M. 50, 172, 180
Ferruci, P. 180
Fineman, S. 180
Firth, J. A. 180
Firth, J. 180
Firth, H., McKeown, P., McIntee,
    J. and Britton, P. 180
Firth, J. A. and Shapiro, D. A. 6,
    172
Fisher, S. 180
Fisher, S. and Reason, J. 180
Flexibility, developing 108
Fluency 105
Focusing 96
Foggo-Pays, E. 180
Fontana, D. 115, 172
Fordham, F. 180
France, R. and Robson, M. 180
Francis, D. and Young, D. 180
Frankl, V. E. 180
French, P. 180
Freud, S. 17
Freudenberger, H. and Richelson,
    G. 180
Fromm, E. 180
Funnelling 139

Gallows humour 87
Geller, L. 180
Gendlin, E. 96, 172
Gendlin, E. T. and Beebe, J. 180
General Adaptation Syndrome 3
George, P. and Kummerow,
    J. 181
Gestalt exercises 67–74
Gestalt therapy 64, 65, 66
Gesture 104
Gibson, R. L. and Mitchell, M.
    H. 181

Gier, M. D., Levick, M. D. and
    Blazina, P. J. 181
Gift of time 39
Gilleard, C. J. 181
Giving permission 29
Goffman, I. 181
Goldberg, L. and Beznitz, S. 181
Gordon, S. and Waldo, M. 181
Gormally, J. 181
Graham, N. M. 181
Ground rules in groups 65
Group
    supervision 167
    support 149–68
Groups, projection in 18
Growth groups 54
Gunning, R. 172
Guru figures 59

Haggerty, L. A. 181
Hales-Tooke, J. 96, 172
Hall, C. 17, 172
Haller, H. 88
Halmos, P. 181
Hamilton, M. S. 181
Hanks, L., Belliston, L. and
    Edwards, D. 181
Hanson, P. 115, 172
Hargie, O., Saunders, C. and
    Dickson, D. 54, 103, 172
Harris, T. 181
Hawkins, P. and Shohet, R. 167,
    172
Health Education Authority 181
Health professional, stress and
    the 1–14
Heins, M., Fahey, S. N. and
    Leiden, L. I. 181
Hemmons, J. 181
Herinck, R. 181
Heron, J. and Reason, P. 145,
    173
Heron, J. 4, 7, 15, 46, 60, 90, 139,
    145, 165, 172
Hewitt, J. 91, 155, 173

Hick, T. D. 173
Hidden area, the 55
Hidden agenda 154
Hindu mantra 95
Hingley, P. and Cooper,
    C. L. 181
Holism 48
Holloway, E. L. 165, 173
Holmes, T. H. and Rahe,
    R. H. 115, 173
Holmes-Rahe Social
    Readjustment scale 115, 116
Holt, R. 181
Hospices 145
Hughes, J. 182
Hull, D. and Schroeder, H. 182
Human Potential Resource
    Group 162
Humanistic therapies 65
Humour, 87
Hurding, R. F. 182
Hutchins, D. E. 182

I–Thou relationship 34
Identification 24
Individuation 39
Inghams, H. 55
Intellectualization 20–1
Intensive care units 145
Intent 104
Interventions, therapeutic 58
Introspection 53
Intuiting 21, 48
Intuitive dimension, the 48
Intuition in counselling 142
Ivey, A. E. 182

Jackins, H. 145, 173
Jacobson, D. 182
Jacobson, S. F. 182
James, M. and Jongeward, D. 182
Jenkins, E. 182
Jenkins, J. F. and Ostchega,
    Y. 182
Jewish mantra 95
Johari window 55, 57

Johnson, D. W. and Johnson, F. P. 182
Jones, J. G., Janman, K., Payne, R. L. and Rick, J. T. 182
Jones, G. 6, 173, 182
Jourard, S. 106, 173
Jung, C. G. 21, 39, 40, 173

Kagan, C. 54, 173
Kahn, R. L. and Cannell, C. F. 139, 173
Kampel, W. and Kampel, M. 182
Kavanagh, K. H. 182
Keller, K. L. and Koenig, W. J. 182
Kelly, C. 182
Kelly, G. 36, 173
Kennedy, E. 182
Kierkegaard, S. 91
Kilty, J. 145, 173
Kim, M. L., McFarland, G. K. and McLane, A. M. 87, 173
Kinasthetic sense 47
Kitzinger, S. 78, 173
Knowles, M. S. et al. 173
Koberg, D. and Bagnal, J. 182
Kopp, S. 182
Kottler, J. A. and Brown, R. W. 183

L'Abate, L. and Milan, M. 183
Lachman, V. D. 183
Laing, R. D. 34, 35, 173
Lang, A. J. and Jakubowski, P. 183
Larson, D. G. 183
Last straw syndrome 24
Lazarus, R. S. and Folkman, S. 183
Le Shan, L. 91, 173
Leading questions 138
Leady, N. K. 183
Leap of faith 91
Learning assertiveness 107
Leech, K. 183
Lennon, M. C. 183

Levine, M. 8, 173
Lewis, H. and Streitfield, H. 183
Lewis, M. 183
Liberman, R. P., King, L. W., DeRisi, W. J. and McCann, M. 183
Life stress assessment 115
Listening 105, 123, 128–32
Listening to the body 50
Literal description 27
Locating feelings in the body 29
Long-term faulty beliefs 23
Lowen, A. 22, 173
Lowen, A. and Lowen, L. 22, 173
Luft, J. 55, 56, 106, 173
Lyon, B. L. and Werner, J. S. 183

Madders, J. 183
Magrath, A., Reid, N. and Boore, J. 183
Management 6
Mantra, using a 94
Margison, F. R. 6, 173
Marshall, E. K. and Kurtz, P. D. 183
Martial arts 50, 55
Maslach, C. 8, 9, 174
Maslow, A. 40, 174
Massage 50
Matthews, D. A., Classen, D. C., Willims, J. L. and Cotton, J. P. 183
May, K. M. 183
McCaffery, M. 78, 174
McCue, J. D. 183
McGuire, J. and Priestley, P. 183
McIntee, J. and Firth, H. 183
Meaning systems 39
Meaning 90
Meaninglessness 88
Meditation 51, 86, 90, 91, 97, 156
Meditation techniques 93–5
Meichembaum, D. and Jaremko, M. E. 184

Meichenbaum, D. 183
Mental mechanisms 17
Merriam, S. 184
Metaphors, use of in
    counselling 128
Meyeroff, J. 174
Middleton, J. F. 184
Milne, D., Burdett, C. and
    Beckett, J. 184
Mind/body 49
Mind/body therapy 22
Mind/body relationship 45
Minimal prompts 42, 129
Model of the self 41
Moore, D. 184
Moreno, J. L. 184
Morris, D. 128, 174
Morsund, J. 184
Moslem mantra 95
Mouton, J. S. and Blake,
    R. R. 184
Muller, P. A. 184
Munro, A., Manthei, B. and
    Small, J. 184
Murgatroyd, S. and Woolfe,
    R. 184
Murgatroyd, S. 132, 174
Murphy, L. R. 184
Murphy, J. M., Nadelson, C. C.
    and Notman, M. T. 184
Murphy, S. A. 184
Muscular pain in stress 21
Myerscough, P. R. 184

Nadler, L. 184
Narnajo, C. and Ornstein,
    R. E. 155, 174
Nash, E. S. 184
Nature of emotions 15
Nature of stress 1
Nausea 33, 88
Need for meaning, the 86
Nelson-Jones, R. 184
Non-linguistic aspects of
    speech 42

Non-verbal aspects of
    communication 128
Noticing the breaths in
    meditation 92
Notman, M. T., Salt, P. and
    Nadelson, C. C. 185
Nutall, P. 185

O'Dowd, T. C. 185
Ohlsen, A. M., Horne, A. M. and
    Lawe, C. F. 185
Onady, A. A., Rodenhauser, P.
    and Market, R. J. 185
Oncology 33, 145
Ontological security 34
Open University Coping With
    Crisis Group 185
Open questions 136
Open area, the 55
Open-ended discussion 156
Organizational stress 102
Osborn, S. M. and Harris,
    G. G. 185
Outer experience of self 42

Pacing 42
Palmer, M. E. and Deck,
    E. S. 185
Paradoxical intention, use of 144
Payne, R. and Firth-Conzens,
    J. 185
Pearce, J. C. 91–3, 174
Pearlin, L. I. 185
Perls, F. 64, 65, 174
Perls, F., Hefferline, R. F. and
    Goodman, P. 75, 174
Personhood, criteria for 37
Phelps, S. and Austin, N. 185
Phenomenology 52
Phillip-Jones, L. 185
Physical aspects of self 38
Physical discomfort 21
Physical tension 76
Physiological responses in stress 3
Pines, A. M., Aronson, E. and
    Kafry, D. 10, 174

Pollack, K. 185
Pope, B. 185
Positive use of emotion 26
Posture 101, 104
Potts, D. 145
Present tense account 28
Preventing stress at work 134
Priestley, P., McQuire, J., Flegg,
    D., Hemsley, V. and
    Welham, D. 185
Problem solving 97, 159
Problems, stress-related 1
Procter, B. D. 185
Professionalism 35
Projection 18–19
Proprioception 47
Proximity to others 44
Psychiatric units 145
Psychoanalysis 64
Psychoanalytical theory 35
Psychoanalytical literature 46
Psychological views of self 35
Psychotherapy 90
Pussyfooting 99–102, 109

Questions 134, 135

Rationalization 19–20
Rawlings, M. E. and Rawlings,
    L. 185
Reaction-formation 20
Reason, P. and Rowan, J. 174
Reddy, M. 185
Redirection 25
Reduced personal
    accomplishment 9
Reductionist theories 36
Reflection 134, 140
Rehearsal 30
Reich, W. 21, 50, 64, 174
Reichian bodywork 50, 55
RELATE (marriage guidance
    council) 63, 123
Relaxation tapes 164
Relaxation
    activities 78–80

response, the 91
scripts 80–84
stress and 76–85
Release of bottled up emotion 27
Remembering 48
Roet, B. 75, 174
Rogers, C. R. 39, 49, 53, 132, 174
Rogers, J. C. and Dodson,
    S. C. 186
Role play 108, 167
Role modelling 107
Rolf, I. 50, 174
Rolfing 50
Roman Catholic mantra 94
Roof-brain chatter 92, 93
Rowan, J. 38, 174
Rushton, A. 6, 174

Sartre, J-P. 35, 33, 41, 88, 174
Scharer, K. 186
Schilling, D. and Poppen, R. 121,
    174
Schmidt, J. A. and Wolfe,
    J. S. 186
Schon, D. A. 186
Schorr, T. M. 186
Schulman, D. 139, 174
Searle, J. 45, 174
Selective reflection 134, 140
Self
    a model of 41
    actualization 40
    and stress 113
    as an instrument 45
    aspects of 36
    conscious use of 45
    outer experience of 42
    monitoring 62
Self-awareness
    activities 62–75
    developing 53
    development, problems in 59
    stress and 98–110
Self-consciousness 51
Self-disclosure 106

Self-exploration 127
Self-image, faulty 22
Self-neglect 7
Selye, H. 3, 174
Sensing 21
Sensing dimension, the 47
Setting unrealistic goals 23
Shafer, P. 186
Shamian, J. and Inhaber, R. 186
Shapiro, E. C., Haseltime, F., and Rowe, M. 186
Shapiro, D. A. 6
Shaw, M. E. 186
Shostak, A. B. 186
Shropshire, C. O. 186
Simon, S. B., Howe, L. W. and Kirschenbaum, H. 186
Singer, P. 175
Sledgehammering 99–102, 109
Smith, E. and Wilks, N. 175
Smith, T. 186
Social aspects of self 38, 41
Socio-cultural aspects of assertiveness 104
Sources of stress 4
Speech, non-linguistic aspects of 42
Speizer, J. J. 186
Spinelli, E. 175
Spiritual distress 87
Spiritual aspects of self 38
Spirituality 86
Sport 55
Steppenwolf 88
Stevens, J. O. 186
Stimulus overload 3
Stimulus-response model of stress 3
Stoll, R. I. 94, 175
Stress
    and feelings 15–30
    and health professionals 5
    and its effects on you 111
    and relaxation 76–85

and self-awareness 32–75, 98–110
and work 111–12
causes of 117
management, workshop on 150
reduction groups 77
values and meditation 86–97
work related 112
workshops 157
Stress reduction, self-awareness and 60
Stress at work, preventing 134
Stress support systems 122–47
Stress-related problems 1
Subpersonalities 38
Supervision in the health professions 149–68
Supervision 164
Support groups 149
Support systems 122–147
Switching 25

Tai chi 55
Taking responsibility 11
Tart, C. 91, 175
Taubman, B. 186
Taylor, S. 186
Taylor, E. 186
Terkel, S. 1, 2, 175
Therapeutic interventions 58
Thinking dimension, the 45
Thinking 21
Thinking aloud 143
Thompson, J. 186
Time, gift of 39
Timing 42, 105
Totton, N. and Edmonston, E. 50, 175
Touch 43
Tough, A. M. 186
Transactional model of stress 3
Transmutation 26
Treat yourself: exercise 91
Trower, P., O'Mahony, J. M. and Dryden, W. 187

Trower, P., Bryant, B. M. and
   Argyle, M. 187
Truax, C. B. and Carkuff,
   R. R. 187

Underlying feelings 29
Unfinished business 154
Unknown area, the 55
Unrealistic goals 23

Value judgements 53, 137
Value-laden questions 138
Values clarification 89
Values clarification
   questionnaire 89, 169–70
Values in stress
   management 86–97
Video taping 55
Views of self, psychological 35
Vingerhoets, A. J. J. M. and
   Marcelissen, F. H. G. 13, 175
Volume of speech 42
Voluntariness in groups 60
Vonnegut, K. 36, 175

Vredenburgh, D. J. and Trinkaus,
   R. J. 187

Wallace, W. A. 187
Wallance, A. 78, 175
Wallis, R. 187
Watkins, J. 187
Weatley, D. 187
Weil, S. W. and McGill, I. 175
Wheeler, D. D. and Janis,
   I. L. 187
Whitaker, D. S. 187
Why? questions 138
Wilkinson, J. and Canter, S. 187
Winn, M. F. 187
Wlodkowski, R. J. 187
Women's groups 54
Woodcock, M. and Frances,
   D. 79, 99, 198, 175
Work related stress 112, 122

Yoga 50, 55

Zander, A. 187
Zastrow, C. 187
Zones of attention 124